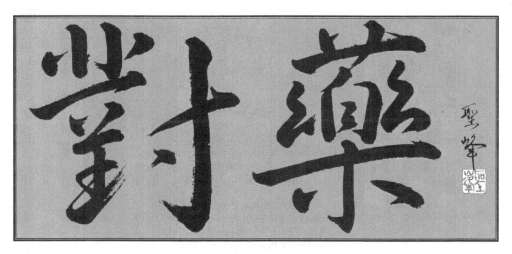

DUI YAO

The Art of Combining
Chinese Medicinals

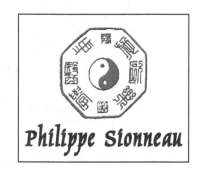

Philippe Sionneau

Translated by Bernard Côté

Blue Poppy Press

Published by:

BLUE POPPY PRESS
A Division of Blue Poppy Enterprises, Inc.
3275-B Prairie Avenue
BOULDER, CO 80301

First Edition, June, 1997
Second Printing, February, 1999
Third Printing, September, 2000
Fourth Printing, April, 2002
Fifth Printing, November, 2003
Sixth Printing, March, 2004
Seventh Printing, February, 2005
Eighth Printing, September, 2005
Ninth Printing, September, 2006
Tenth Printing, May, 2007
Eleventh Printing, May, 2008
Twelveth Printing, June, 2009
Thirteenth Printing, September, 2010
Fourteenth Printing, September 2011
Fifteenth Printing, June, 2013
Sixteenth Printing, September, 2014
Seventeenth Printing, June, 2015
Eighteenth Printing, May, 2016
Nineteenth Printing, December, 2016

ISBN 0-936185-81-3
ISBN 978-0-936185-81-1

COMP Designation: Original work using a standard translational terminology

20 19

Printed at Edwards Brothers Malloy, Ann Arbor, MI

Cover calligraphy by Michael Sullivan (Seiho)
Cover design by Eric J. Brearton

Printed on recycled paper with soy inks

Dedication

For Pierre, my father, and through him, to all my family lineage. Respect, love, and gratitude.

"It is more useful to light a small lamp than to curse the darkness." *Lao Zi*

Editor's Preface

This book is about the art of combining Chinese medicinals. The study of such Chinese medicinal combinations is an intermediary step between memorizing the Chinese materia medica as single ingredients and memorizing formulas as a whole. By studying such two medicinal combinations, one can more easily understand and remember why formulas are composed as they are. In addition, such two medicinal combinations are very important when it comes to modifying standard formulas with additions and subtractions. In Chinese medicine, it is typical to add two medicinals to address any complicating patterns or any particular signs and symptoms. This allows such modifications to be more powerful and more precise. And lastly, the study of such combinations serves as a basis for creating new formulas from scratch. Therefore, the study of two medicinal combinations is an important part of studying so-called Chinese herbal medicine, a part which has previously been overlooked by the English language Chinese literature.

The combinations in this book have all been empirically tested, in many cases for at least two thousand years. It is these combinations that the practitioner can rest assured are the effective ones. When one looks at the temperatures, natures, functions, and indications of two medicinals, one may think that, theoretically, they should work well together for a certain purpose. However, in actual clinical fact, maybe they do and maybe they do not. Over not less than two hundred generations of literate, professional practitioners, Chinese doctors have identified those combinations which are, in fact, the most effective. By studying and using such a core repertoire of empirically effective combinations, one can more quickly make progress in their study and practice of Chinese herbal medicine.

Using this book

In attempting to use this book, the reader will see that the author emphasizes the very precise distinction between medicinals, varieties of medicinals, methods of prepartion, and dosages. In particular, he often stipulates that for certain purposes, a certain prepared form of a medicinal should be used. For instance, he may specify uncooked or dry *Jiang* (Rhizoma Zingiberis) or uncooked or honey mix-fried *Huang Qi* (Radix Astragali Membranacei). In Chinese, the preparation of medicinals is called *pao zhi* and, in China, the study of such methods of preparation and their clinical use is a standard part of every Chinese medical practitioner's undergraduate training. Since this is also an aspect of Chinese medicine that has been largely overlooked in the West, the reader is referred to Philippe Sionneau's companion volume, *Pao Zhi: An Introduction to the Use of Processed Chinese Medicinals* also published by Blue Poppy Press, for information on the methods and indications of processed medicinals suggested in this book. When one combines the right medicinals which have been processed in the right way, one truly has a refined and clinically effective treatment.

The reader will also see that this book has been designed in tabular fashion to allow the quicker and easier comparison of the properties of individual medicinals within a pair. In the section titled "Major Indications of the Combination", the reader will find numbers in parentheses after some of these indications. These numbers then appear below in the section titled "Notes" where the author explains something further vis a vis these particular indications. Below these numbered notes, there may also be letters of the alphabet in parentheses as well. These alphabetized notes do not relate in a specific way to any of the previous indications. Rather, they are more generalized notes about different varieties of the same medicinal or discussions of dosages, special cautions, toxicity, etc.

About this book

This book is a special English language version of Philippe Sionneau's *Pharmacopee Chinoise: L'art des associations (Chinese Pharmacopea: The Art of Combinations)*. By that, I mean that it is not exactly a translation. The process of creation of this book began with Bernard Cote of Montreal translating *Pharmacopee Chinoise* into English. However, during the editing process, it became clear that the needs of English reading practitioners of Chinese medicine are not the same as those of French reading practitioners.

At Blue Poppy Press, we are very concerned with the accuracy of the translation and transmission of technical material from its Chinese sources. This material is meant to be put into practice in a very precise manner, and if one prescribes the wrong medicinals because of an error in translation, this can have disasterous results for the patient and eventually for the profession. Therefore, Blue Poppy Press has adopted Nigel Wiseman's English terminology, as appearing in *English-Chinese Chinese-English Dictionary of Chinese Medicine*, Hunan Science & Technology Press, Changhsa, 1995, for the translation of technical Chinese medical terms. In addition, we favor a denotative translation with commentaries or footnotes over a connotative translation. Thus, in the creation of this book, we were faced with the special problems of going from French to English *after* the author had gone from Chinese to French without the aid of such a linguistically accurate Chinese-French Chinese medical dictionary.

That meant that after Bernard was finished translating the French into English and I was finished editing his English, the manuscript was then sent back to Philippe for him to rectify all the technical terms and make them corresponds to Nigel's as far as possible. Therefore, if one compares the original French version with this English endition, one will see some changes in the text. For instance, instead of saying "dispels blood stasis" as does the French, our version reads, "dispels stasis", since this is Nigel's translation of the original Chinese treatment principles. Other changes in this English language version are that we have deleted the preface to the French addition and we also left out those parts of Philippe's book which appear in his other books already published by Blue Poppy Press.

Medicinal identifications used in this book are mostly based on the second, revised edition of Bensky & Gamble's *Chinese Herbal Medicine: Materia Medica*, Eastland Press, Seattle, 1993. However, rather than putting the Latinate pharmocological names first, we have placed the Pinyin transliteration of the Chinese names first, similar to how we identify acupuncture points. Formula names are our own translations.

It is our great pleasure to be able to share the knoweldge and research of such a Western practitioner of Chinese medicine as Philippe Sionneau. Philippe has made and we feel confident will continue to make an important contribution to the Western Chinese medical literature. We hope that this book will help Western practitioners more accurately and effectively combine Chinese medicinals in their prescriptions.

Bob Flaws
Boulder, CO

Translator's Preface

The translation into English of a text written in French and pertaining to Chinese medicine doubly underscores the challenge for Westerners in grasping the complexity and depth of traditional Chinese medical thinking. It is with an awareness of this dimension that this work has been translated. Hopefully, the reader will draw from their own knowledge to widen and deepen the possibilities of this translation. It is with this perspective that a real interaction may occur between the Chinese source text, the author of this work, Philippe Sionneau, the translator, and, most important of all, the reader who will really complete this project by integrating the knowledge contained herein into their clinical practice.

The colossal achievement of Philippe Sionneau and his contribution to the Chinese medical literature published in the West is obvious from the very first pages of this book. The complexity of the theoretical concepts becomes a source of insight and inspiration under his pen. His endeavor to familiarize Western practitioners with the comparative aspects of Chinese medicinals will grow in a multitude of applications in clinical practice.

Bernard Côté
Montréal

Contents

1

The Art of Combining Chinese Medicinal Substances: Its Theory, Methodology & Advantages

Within the Chinese materia medica, there are numerous combinations of two medicinals used together. Each of these pairs of medicinals is known to be especially effective for the treatment of specific pathological conditions. Based on empirical experience, these combinations' therapeutic effect is safe, consistent, and should not be ignored by Western practitioners of Chinese medicine. Below are the main ways in which combinations of medicinals are described and applied in Chinese medicine.

A. Combining to enhance mutual complementarity

Some medicinal substances complement each other in a harmonious and balanced way, reinforcing each other's therapeutic action.

1. Medicinal substances of the same type which complement each other

Medicinal substances from the same class have a tendency to complement and enhance each other. This is the most common type of medicinal combining seen in Chinese medicine. Nevertheless, some pairs are more effective and better known than others. For example:

Ma Huang (Herba Ephedrae) & Gui Zhi (Ramulus Cinnamomi Cassiae)

Ma Huang scatters cold and strongly resolves the exterior (*i.e.*, promotes sweating). *Gui Zhi* dispels wind and moderately resolves the exterior. When combined together, they powerfully resolve the exterior. In other words, their action is drastic.

Da Huang (Radix Et Rhizoma Rhei) & Mang Xiao (Mirabilitum)

Da Huang drains fire, cools the blood, and frees the flow of the stools.[1] *Mang Xiao* drains heat, moistens dryness, and softens the stools. When combined together, *Mang Xiao* softens the stools and *Da Huang* precipitates them. This combination, therefore, effectively treats constipation with hard dry stools due to replete heat in the stomach and intestines.

---

[1] Wiseman translates *tong bian* as free the stool. We have added the word flow to emphasize the implied effect on the movement of the stool.

Shi Gao (Gypsum Fibrosum) & *Zhi Mu* (Rhizoma Anemarrhenae Aspheloidis)

Shi Gao clears heat from the qi division and drains fire. *Zhi Mu* nourishes yin and downbears fire. When combined together, they clear and strongly drain replete heat while protecting fluids and humors.

2. Medicinal substances of different types which complement each other

Frequently, medicinals of very different types are used together since they complement each other in an ideal way in order to treat a very specific imbalance. For example:

a) To treat root (*ben*) and branch (*biao*) simultaneously

Dang Shen (Radix Codonopsitis Pilosulae) & *Zi Su Ye* (Folium Perillae Frutescentis)

Dang Shen fortifies the spleen and supplements the qi. *Zi Su Ye* resolves the exterior, thus promoting sweating. Together, they supplement the qi while resolving the exterior. One supports the correct qi and treats the root, while the other drains the evil qi and treats the branch. This combination is particularly suitable for cases of acute cold with enduring qi vacuity.

b) To supplement two divisions (qi & blood) simultaneously

Huang Qi (Radix Astragali Membranacei) & *Dang Gui* (Radix Angelicae Sinensis)

Huang Qi supplements the spleen and boosts the qi in order to engender and transform the blood. *Dang Gui* nourishes the blood, quickens the blood, and harmonizes the blood. When combined together, they supplement the qi and blood simultaneously in cases of qi and blood dual vacuity.

c) To treat two different pathological situations simultaneously

Chuan Lian Zi (Fructus Meliae Toosendan) & *Yan Hu Suo* (Rhizoma Corydalis Yanhusuo)

Chuan Lian Zi is cold. It clears heat, moves the qi, soothes the liver, and stops pain. *Yan Hu Suo* is warm. It quickens the blood, moves the qi, and stops pain. When combined together, they move the qi and blood and treat pain due to qi stagnation and blood stasis in either a cold or heat pattern.

d) To harmonize the exterior & interior

Chai Hu (Radix Bupleuri) & *Huang Qin* (Radix Scutellariae Baicalensis)

Chai Hu drains evil qi in the exterior in a *shao yang* pattern, while *Huang Qin* drains evil qi in the interior in a *shao yang* pattern. Together, they harmonize the *shao yang*.

e) To supplement & drain simultaneously

Huang Qi (Radix Astragali Membranacei) & *Fang Feng* (Radix Ledebouriellae Divaricatae)

Huang Qi supplements the qi and fortifies the spleen, upbears yang, secures the exterior, and stops sweating. *Fang Feng* dispels wind, resolves the exterior, and dispels wind dampness. When combined together, one supplements and the other dispels. They secure the exterior defensive at the same time as draining external evils from the exterior.

f) To reinforce an action

Cang Zhu (Rhizoma Atractylodis) & *Huang Bai* (Cortex Phellodendri)

Cang Zhu fortifies the spleen, dries dampness, and dispels wind dampness. *Huang Bai* clears heat, drains vacuity heat, and dries dampness in the lower burner. When combined together, one effectively dries and the other effectively clears. Thus, when combined together, they effectively clear heat and dry dampness in the lower burner.

B. Combining opposites to enhance complementarity

Medicinal substances of different natures have different and even opposite functions and effects. It is sometimes useful to use these oppositions to produce a particular therapeutic action which cannot be obtained by using medicinals of the same type.

1. Combining cold & hot natured medicinals

Cold-natured and hot-natured medicinals commonly have opposite functions which are often difficult to reconcile. Nevertheless, when well selected and in the right dosage, they can be used together without problem and generate remarkable therapeutic effects. For example:

Shi Gao (Gypsum Fibrosum) & *Gui Zhi* (Ramulus Cinnamomi Cassiae)

Shi Gao is very cold. Its tropism is for the qi division.[2] It clears and drains heat from the *yang ming* and from the muscles (dosage important). *Gui Zhi* is warm, resolves the exterior, and scatters cold. Together, one is cold, the other is warm. Therefore, this combination is cool without producing congelation and stasis (which cold might otherwise be expected to cause). In addition, it is warm without being drying (which heat might otherwise be expected to cause). When combined together, they clear heat, free the flow of the network vessels, and treat heat impediment or *bi* (*i.e.*, hot, red, swollen, and painful joints).

Huang Lian (Rhizoma Coptidis Chinensis) & *Wu Zhu Yu* (Fructus Evodiae Rutecarpae)

Huang Lian is bitter and cold. It clears heat, dries dampness, and drains heart, liver, and stomach fire. *Wu Zhu Yu* is acrid and warm. It downbears counterflowing stomach qi and stops vomiting, soothes the liver and stops pain. Together, one is cold, the other is hot. They soothe the liver and drain heat from the liver and stomach while treating vomiting, acid regurgitation, and lateral costal pain.

2. Simultaneous supplementation & drainage

Supplementation is a treatment method aimed at supporting the correct qi. Draining is a treatment method which aims at eliminating evil qi. In some cases, it is necessary to support the correct qi and drain the evil qi simultaneously when a repletion (*i.e.*, an acute condition) manifests at the same time there is a vacuity

---

[2]   Wiseman translates *fen* as aspect. The character shows a knife dividing something into two pieces. Therefore, we believe the word division is more accurate and is a better denotative translation while conveying in English the exact same connotation as the word aspect.

(*i.e.*, enduring condition) already present or when vacuity and repletion coexist in the same pattern. For example:

Da Huang (Radix Et Rhizoma Rhei) & Ren Shen (Radix Panacis Ginseng)

Da Huang is bitter and cold. It attacks evils. *Ren Shen* is sweet and neutral. It strongly supplements the original qi. When combined together, they support the correct qi while draining evils when there is accumulation in the large intestine in an elderly or weak person.

Huang Lian (Rhizoma Coptidis Chinensis) & E Jiao (Gelatinum Corii Asini)

Huang Lian is bitter and cold. It clears and drains heart fire, and clears and dries damp heat. Its function is to drain evil heat. *E Jiao* is sweet and neutral. It nourishes yin and blood. Its function is to support the correct qi. When combined together, they drain replete fire and supplement and enrich yin vacuity. This combination is used in cases of warm disease which damages yin and causes insomnia and/or vexation and agitation or in cases of dysentery of the heat type which damages yin accompanied by pus and blood in the stools.

Zhi Shi (Fructus Immaturus Citri Aurantii) & Bai Zhu (Rhizoma Atractylodis Macrocephalae)

Zhi Shi breaks qi stagnation and disperses food accumulation. *Bai Zhu* fortifies the spleen and reinforces the functions of movement and transformation of the middle burner. When combined together, they treat food stagnation (*i.e.*, repletion) due to spleen vacuity.

3. Opening & gathering simultaneously

This is a treatment method similar to simultaneous supplementation and drainage. However, its therapeutic effects aim at regulating the movement of qi by normalizing qi counterflow (*i.e.*, lung, stomach, and/or liver qi counterflow) and by reinforcing the correct movement of qi (*i.e.* the diffusion and descent of lung qi, the descent of stomach qi, the upbearing of spleen qi, and the reception of qi by the kidneys). For example:

Xi Xin (Herba Asari Cum Radice) & Wu Wei Zi (Fructus Schisandrae Chinensis)

Xi Xin is acrid and warm and effuses and scatters wind cold. It warms the lungs and transforms phlegm cold. *Xi Xin* effuses and opens. *Wu Wei Zi* is acrid and warm and supplements the lungs and kidneys. It constrains the lung qi. *Wu Wei Zi* supplements and gathers. When combined together, these two medicinals effuse and scatter wind cold which causes lung qi blockage. At the same time, they constrain the lung qi which tends to counterflow. Thus they stop cough and calm asthma.[3] In the presence of wind cold, lung qi is blocked by the external evils, and the diffusion and descent of the lung qi is disturbed. The treatment principle consists of effusing and scattering wind cold, diffusing the lungs, and allowing perfusion of the qi. This is the role of *Xi Xin*. If there is cough or asthma, lung qi counterflows upward. If the affection is

---

[3]   Wiseman gives calm for *ping*. While that is an acceptable connotative translation, the reader should know that the character literally means to level. This spatial dimension is important for understanding when and why one calms asthma or calms the liver. In other words, calming is used when one levels upwardly counterflowing qi.

severe or prolonged, this tends to damage the lung qi. The treatment principle consists then of regulating the lung qi and constraining the lung qi. This is the role of *Wu Wei Zi*.

4. Combining fixed (*shou*) & travelling (*zou*) characteristics

The notions of *zou* and *shou* are difficult to translate. *Zou* indicates that a medicinal substance tends to be active, mobile, that it tends to move, that it can penetrate easily every minute part of the system, or that it can direct itself toward the exterior or into and through the channels easily. *Shou*, on the other hand, indicates that a medicinal substance tends to have a contracting action, that it works locally, and that it is fixed and tranquil and without any major qi transformation. Such medicinals tend to have an astringent property, the property of firming, protecting, supplementing, alleviating or pacifying.

These characteristics are always relative and not absolute. Therefore, a medicinal can be fixed in relation to one substance, and mobile in relation to another. It is easier to grasp these notions by studying the effects of *Sheng Huang Qi* (uncooked Radix Astragali Membranacei) and *Mi Zhi Huang Qi* (honey mix-fried Radix Astragali Membranacei).

Uncooked *Huang Qi* has a light property. Its flavor is slightly sweet and its nature is slightly warm. It tends to be mobile (*zou*). Its mobile character allows it to:

a. Direct itself towards the exterior, stop perspiration, and secure the defensive qi
b. Direct itself into the channels and treat the sequelae of hemiplegia
c. Direct itself towards the joints and treat impediment (*i.e., bi*)
d. Direct itself towards the skin and treat dermatological conditions

Honey mix-fried *Huang Qi* has a heavy property. It is very sweet in flavor and warm in nature. It tends to be fixed (*shou*). Its fixed character directs its action towards the interior, concentrating and fixing its action in the middle burner, allowing it to:

a. Supplement spleen and stomach qi
b. Upbear the clear yang of the middle burner

This method consists of combining "fixed" and "mobile" medicinals in order to reinforce a particular therapeutic action. For example:

Hua Shi (Talcum) & Zhi Gan Cao (mix-fried Radix Glycyrrhizae)

Hua Shi is sweet and cold and has a "slippery" nature. It downbears the lung qi, drains summerheat, eliminates vexation and agitation, opens the orifices, and disinhibits urination. It is a "mobile" substance. *Zhi Gan Cao* is sweet and neutral and supplements the qi, harmonizes and tempers the action of other medicinals, relieves tension, and stops pain. It is a "fixed" substance. When combined together, *Zhi Gan Cao* tempers the drastic action of *Hua Shi*. Together, they clear heat, drain summerheat, and disinhibit urination without damaging the middle burner.

Dang Gui (Radix Angelicae Sinensis) & *Bai Shao* (Radix Albus Paeoniae Lactiflorae)

Dang Gui is sweet, acrid, and warm. It supplements the blood, quickens the blood, regulates menstruation, and stops pain. Its nature is "mobile." It quickens the blood due to its acrid, moving nature. *Bai Shao* is bitter, sour, and slightly cold. It nourishes the blood, constrains yin, emolliates the liver, and stops pain. Its "fixed" character constrains yin due to its astringent nature. Together, one is mobile, the other fixed. Thus they regulate the blood efficiently.

5. To downbear & upbear simultaneously

This method consists of regulating the upbearing and downbearing of the qi. For example:

Jie Geng (Radix Platycodi Grandiflori) & *Zhi Ke* (Fructus Citri Aurantii)

Jie Geng is bitter, acrid, and neutral. It diffuses the lung qi and transforms phlegm. It promotes ascending movement and directs the action of other medicinals toward the upper part of the body. *Zhi Ke* is bitter and slightly cold. It moves the qi, opens the center, and disperses distention. It promotes descending movement. Together, one upbears, the other downbears. When combined together, they regulate the movement of qi and loosen the chest and diaphragm. Therefore, they treat chest and diaphragm distention due to phlegm accumulation.

Hua Shi (Talcum) & *He Ye* (Folium Nelumbinis Nuciferae)

Hua Shi clears summerheat and eliminates dampness, drains heat and downbears turbid yin. *He Ye* eliminates summerheat, clears heat, and upbears clear yang. When combined together, one upbears, the other downbears. Together, they upbear the clear and downbear the turbid. Thus, they drain summerheat and eliminate dampness efficiently.

C. Combining in order to protect

Some medicinal substances tend to damage the stomach qi because of their too drastic action. The stomach is the source of transformation of food and thus is the source of the transformation and engenderment of the qi, blood, and latter heaven (*i.e.*, acquired) essence. Therefore, an imbalance of this organ will directly affect the health of the individual. Hence, it is important to alleviate and eliminate the secondary effects of such drastic medicinals and to protect the stomach qi. For example:

Ci Shi (Magnetite) & *Shen Qu* (Massa Medica Fermentata)

Ci Shi is acrid and cold and has heavy characteristics. It quiets the spirit and calms the heart, nourishes the kidneys and brightens the eyes. It also levels (or calms) the liver and subdues yang. Magnetite is a mineral which is hard to assimilate and demands a particular effort from the stomach. *Shen Qu* is sweet, acrid, and warm. It disperses food accumulation and harmonizes the stomach. It facilitates the assimilation of minerals and protects the stomach. When combined together, *Shen Qu* allows the person to benefit from the properties of *Ci Shi* without damaging the stomach qi.

Shi Gao (Gypsum Fibrosum) & *Geng Mi* (Semen Oryzae Sativae)

Shi Gao is acrid, sweet, and cold. It drains the muscles and clears heat. *Geng Mi* is sweet and neutral. It regulates and protects the stomach qi against medicinals of a very cold nature. When combined together, *Geng Mi* allows the person to benefit from the properties of *Shi Gao* without damaging stomach yang.

Ting Li Zi (Semen Lepidii) & *Da Zao* (Fructus Zizyphi Jujubae)

Ting Li Zi is acrid and draining, bitter and draining, cold and inwardly lowering. It drains the lungs and calms asthma. *Da Zao* is sweet, warm, and harmonizing. It moderates the drastic action of *Ting Li Zi*, protecting lung and stomach qi and yin. When combined together, *Da Zao* allows the person to benefit from the proprieties of *Ting Li Zi* without it damaging the lungs and stomach.

D. Combining in order to harmonize

Some medicinals are often prescribed to balance, reconcile, and make coherent the simultaneous action of other medicinals. These harmonizing medicinals all have a sweet flavor. This flavor is associated with the earth phase which is harmonizing and centering and which is a reference point around which the other phases spread and interact.

Harmonizing medicinals

Zhi Gan Cao (mix-fried Radix Glycyrrhizae)

Functions: *Zhi Gan Cao* balances the actions of many medicinals. For example, it lessens the warming action of *Gan Jiang* (dry Rhizoma Zingiberis) and *Fu Zi* (Radix Lateralis Praeparatus Aconiti Carmichaeli) and preserves yin. It tempers the cooling action of *Shi Gao* (Gypsum Fibrosum) and *Zhi Mu* (Rhizoma Anemarrhenae Aspheloidis) and protects the stomach. It lessens the precipitating or purging action of *Da Huang* (Radix Et Rhizoma Rhei) and *Mang Xiao* (Mirabilitum) and protects the correct qi. It tempers the supplementing action of *Dang Shen* (Radix Codonopsitis Pilosulae), *Huang Qi* (Radix Astragali Membranacei), *Dang Dui* (Radix Angelicae Sinensis), and *Shu Di Huang* (cooked Radix Rehmanniae) and allows for the prolonged use of supplements. It reconciles substances having opposite actions or natures, such as *Gan Jiang* and *Huang Lian* (Rhizoma Coptidis Chinensis).

Caution: In case of edema, oliguria, anuria, or hypertension, the use of *Zhi Gan Cao* and *Gan Cao* must be reduced and short in duration. In case of edema and oliguria, *Gan Cao Shao* (Extremitas Radicis Glycyrrhizae) can be prescribed. In all of these cases, *Gan Cao* can be replaced by *Da Zao* (Fructus Zizyphi Jujubae).

Gan Cao (Radix Glycyrrhizae)

Functions: This medicinal has identical properties to *Zhi Gan Cao* but is used with heat patterns.

Da Zao (Fructus Zizyphi Jujubae)

Functions: Harmonizes the actions of other medicinals. However, it is less effective than *Zhi Gan Cao*. It is used when *Zhi Gan Cao* is incompatible with certain other medicinals, such as *Gan Sui* (Radix Euphorbiae Kansui), *Yuan Hua* (Flos Daphnis Genkwae), *Jing Da Ji* (Radix Euphorbiae Pekinensis), and *Hai Zao* (Herba Sargassii), or in case of edema, anuria, and hypertension. It protects the middle burner and stomach when the action of certain medicinals are drastic, for example, *Ting Li Zi* (Semen Lepidii). Together with *Sheng Jiang* (uncooked Rhizoma Zingiberis), it harmonizes the constructive and defensive qi.

Feng Mi (Honey)

Functions: Honey harmonizes the action of other medicinals and lessens the toxicity of *Fu Zi* (Radix Lateralis Praeparatus Aconiti Carmichaeli) and *Wu Tou* (Radix Aconiti Carmichaeli).

E. Combining to guide

Messenger medicinals allow the leading of the action of other medicinals towards very precise areas of the body in order to exert their effect at the site of the imbalance or its pathological manifestations. These ambassadors specify, refine, reinforce, and even transform the impact of a therapeutic effect. Adding such a messenger medicinal to a prescription adapts that prescription more precisely to the situation at hand and makes it more effective in clinical practice. Thus it is said in Chinese, "*Yao wu yin shi, ze bu tong bing suo* (Medicinal substances without guides cannot reach the site of the illness)." For example:

Sheng Ma (Rhizoma Cimicifugae)

Functions: This medicinal guides the action of other medicinals towards the *yang ming* bowels. In terms of the stomach, it helps treat toothache, oral ulcers, and stomatitis. In terms of the large intestine, it helps to treat constipation. Cimicifuga also guides the action of medicinals towards the upper part of the body (*i.e.*, the head and face).

Jie Geng (Radix Platycodi Grandiflori)

Functions: This medicinal guides the action of other medicinals towards the lungs and chest. It raises towards the middle burner the action of medicinals usually addressing the lower burner. For example, in *Shen Ling Bai Zhu San* (Ginseng, Poria & Atractylodes Powder), *Jie Geng* guides the action of *Yi Yi Ren* (Semen Coicis Lachryma-jobi), *Lian Zi* (Semen Nelumbinis Nuciferae), and *Shan Yao* (Radix Dioscoreae Oppositae) from the lower to the middle burner.

Huai Niu Xi (Radix Achyranthis Bidentatae) & **Chuan Niu Xi** (Radix Cyathulae Officinalis)

Functions: Both *Huai Niu Xi* and *Chuan Niu Xi* guide the blood to move towards the lower part of the body. Thus, they treat bleeding in the upper part of the body, such as hematemesis and epistaxis. They downbear vacuity heat in the upper part of the body manifesting such symptoms as oral ulcers, glossitis, toothache, and sore throat. And they guide the action of other medicinals toward the lower part of the body to treat diseases located below the knees.

Chai Hu (Radix Bupleuri)

Functions: This medicinal guides the action of other medicinals to the liver and gallbladder channels. It guides the action of other medicinals to the upper part of the body (*i.e.*, the head and face). And it guides the action of other medicinals to the lateral costal region.

Gua Lou Pi (Pericarpium Trichosanthis Kirlowii)

Functions: This medicinal guides the action of other medicinals to the chest.

Qin Jiao (Radix Gentianae Macrophyllae)

Functions: This medicinal guides the action of other medicinals to the spine and lumbar area.

Jiang Huang (Rhizoma Curcumae Longae)

Functions: This medicinal guides the action of other medicinals to the upper extremities and shoulders.

Wu Zhu Yu (Fructus Evodiae Rutecarpae)

Functions: This medicinal guides the action of other medicinals to the liver channel. At a certain dosage, it reinforces the action of other medicinals which clear liver fire, treat acid vomiting, or treat *jue yin* headaches.

Rou Gui (Cortex Cinnamomi Cassiae)

Functions: Returns yang (fire) to its lower source in the treatment of sore throat, oral ulcers, glossitis, and other such symptoms of floating yang.

Ma Huang (Herba Ephedrae)

Functions: This medicinal guides the action of other medicinals to the exterior and the skin in the treatment of various types of dermatoses.

Di Long (Lumbricus), *Chuan Shan Jia* (Squama Manitis Pentadactylis) & *Luo Shi Tang* (Caulis Trachelospermi)

Functions: These medicinals guide the action of other medicinals towards the channels and network vessels as well as towards the muscles and sinews in the treatment of paralysis, impediment, sinew or muscle pain, and obstructions of the channels.

Guiding Medicinals	
Channel Destinations	**Messenger Medicinals**
Hand *Tai Yang* Small Intestine	*Mu Tong* (Caulis Akebiae) *Deng Xin Cao* (Medulla Junci Effusi) *Gao Ben* (Radix Et Rhizoma Ligustici Chinensis) *Huang Bai* (Cortex Phellodendri)
Foot *Tai Yang* Bladder	*Ge Gen* (Radix Puerariae) *Qiang Huo* (Radix Et Rhizoma Notopterygii)
Hand *Yang Ming* Large Intestine	*Da Huang* (Radix Et Rhizoma Rhei) *Bai Zhi* (Radix Angelicae Dahuricae) *Sheng Ma* (Rhizoma Cimicifugae) *Shi Gao* (Gypsum Fibrosum)
Foot *Yang Ming* Stomach	*Bai Zhi* (Radix Angelicae Dahuricae) *Sheng Ma* (Rhizoma Cimicifugae) *Shi Gao* (Gypsum Fibrosum) *Ge Gen* (Radix Puerariae)
Hand *Shao Yang* Triple Burner	Upper Burner: *Zhi Zi* (Fructus Gardeniae Jasminoidis) *Gui Zhi* (Ramulus Cinnamomi Cassiae) *Wan Qian* (Fructus Forsythiae Suspensae) *Di Gu Pu* (Cortex Radicis Lycii Chinensis) Middle Burner: *Qing Pi* (Pericarpium Citri Reticulatae Viride) Lower Burner: *Fu Zi* (Radix Lateralis Praeparatus Aconiti Carmichaeli)
Foot *Shao Yang* Gallbladder	*Chai Hu* (Radix Bupleuri) *Qing Pi* (Pericarpium Citri Reticulatae Viride)
Hand *Tai Yin* Lungs	*Jie Geng* (Radix Platycodi Grandiflori) *Sheng Ma* (Radix Cimicifugae) *Cang Bai* (Bulbus Allii Fistulosi) *Bai Zhi* (Radix Angelicae Dahuricae)
Foot *Tai Yin* Spleen	*Bai Zhu* (Radix Atractylodis Macrocephalae) *Ge Gen* (Radix Puerariae) *Cang Zhu* (Rhizoma Atractylodis) *Sheng Ma* (Rhizoma Cimicifugae) *Bai Shao* (Radix Albus Paeoniae Lactiflorae)
Hand *Shao Yin* Heart	*Huang Lian* (Rhizoma Coptidis Chinensis) *Xi Xin* (Herba Asari Cum Radice)
Foot *Shao Yin* Kidney	*Du Huo* (Radix Angelicae Pubescentis) *Rou Gui* (Cortex Cinnamomi Cassiae) *Zhi Mu* (Rhizoma Anemarrhenae Aspheloidis) *Xi Xin* (Herba Asari Cum Radice)

Hand *Jue Yin* Pericardium	*Chai Hu* (Radix Bupleuri) *Mu Dan* (Cortex Radicis Moutan)
Foot *Jue Yin* Liver	*Wu Zhu Yu* (Fructus Evodiae Rutecarpae) *Chai Hu* (Radix Bupleuri) *Chuan Xiong* (Radix Ligustici Wallichii) *Qing Pi* (Pericarpium Citri Reticulatae Viride)

F. Combining flavors & natures

At a high level of mastery, one not only prescribes Chinese medicinals based on their clinical indication, but also combines and prescribes medicinals according to their flavors and natures. In that case, one not only thinks in terms of medicinals' indications but in term of the movement of qi and their thermic effect. These effects are produced by the combination of medicinals' flavors and natures in the human body. At this level, Chinese medicine then becomes truly subtle art. Below are mentioned only some famous such combinations without elaborating on their underlying mechanisms. Such a discourse would constitute an entire treatise on flavors and natures.

Acrid + sweet = draining

    Example: *Ma Huang* (Herba Ephedrae) + *Zhi Gan Cao* (mix-fried Radix Glycyrrhizae)

Acrid + sweet = supplementing & engendering yang

    Example: *Gui Zhi* (Ramulus Cinnamomi Cassiae) + *Yi Tang* (Saccharum Granorum)

Acrid + sweet + warm = upbearing yang

    Example: *Huang Qi* (Radix Astragali Membranacei) + *Sheng Ma* (Rhizoma Cimicifugae)

Acrid + sweet + warm = arousing of the spleen & transforming phlegm

    Example: *Gan Jiang* (dry Rhizoma Zingiberis) + *Fu Ling* (Sclerotium Poriae Cocos)

Acrid + bland + warm = stimulating the bladder's qi mechanism & disinhibiting urination

    Example: *Gui Zhi* (Ramulus Cinnamomi Cassiae) + *Fu Ling* (Sclerotium Poriae Cocos)

Acrid + astringent = draining & securing simultaneously

    Example: *Xi Xin* (Herba Asari Cum Rradice) + *Wu Wei Zi* (Fructus Schisandrae Chinensis)

Acrid + warm = dispelling wind cold

    Example: *Gui Zhi* (Ramulus Cinnamomi Cassiae) + *Ma Huang* (Herba Ephedrae)

Acrid + cool = clearing heat & dispelling wind heat

    Example: *Dan Dou Chi* (Semen Praeparatus Sojae) + *Bo He(* Herba Menthae Haplocalycis)

Acrid + cold = clearing heat & draining fire

Example: *Shi Gao* (Gypsum Fibrosum) + *Zhu Ye* (Folium Bambusae)

Acrid + hot = warming the center & returning yang

Example: *Gan Jiang* (dry Rhizoma Zingiberis) + *Fu Zi* (Radix Lateralis Praeparatus Aconiti Carmichaeli)

Acrid + hot = warming yang, dissipating cold, eliminating obstruction & stopping pain

Example: *Gui Zhi* (Ramulus Cinnamomi Cassiae) + *Fu Zi* (Radix Lateralis Praeparatus Aconiti Carmichaeli)

Bitter + acrid = moving, opening & downbearing

Example: *Zi Su Ye* (Folium Perillae Frutescentis) + *Huang Lian* (Rhizoma Coptidis Chinensis)

Bitter + cold = clearing heat, draining fire & resolving toxins

Example: *Huang Qin* (Radix Scutellariae Baicalensis) + *Huang Lian* (Rhizoma Coptidis Chinensis)

Bitter + cold = drying dampness & clearing heat

Example: *Cang Zhu* (Rhizoma Atractylodis) + *Huang Bai* (Cortex Phellodendri)

Bitter + cold = draining fire & hardening yin

Example: *Huang Bai* (Cortex Phellodendri) + *Zhi Mu* (Rhizoma Anemarrhenae Aspheloidis)

Bitter + salty + cold = softening & emolliating, precipitating heat accumulations

Example: *Da Huang* (Radix Et Rhizoma Rhei) + *Mang Xiao* (Mirabilitum)

Bitter + salty = draining fire & softening the hard

Example: *Xia Ku Cao* (Spica Prunellae Vulgaris) + *Mu Li* (Concha Ostreae)

Bitter + warm = drying cold dampness

Example: *Cang Zhu* (Rhizoma Atractylodis) + *Hou Po* (Cortex Magnoliae Officinalis)

Bitter + hot = precipitation of cold accumulations

Example: *Da Huang* (Radix Et Rhizoma Rhei) + *Fu Zi* (Radix Lateralis Praeparatus Aconiti Carmichaeli)

Sweet + bland = percolating dampness & disinhibiting urination

Example: *Fu Ling* (Sclerotium Poriae Cocos) + *Yi Yi Ren* (Semen Coicis Lachryma-jobi)

Sweet + warm = supplementing the center & boosting the qi

Example: *Dang Shen* (Radix Codonopsitis Pilosulae) + *Huang Qi* (Radix Astragali Membranacei)

Sweet + warm = abating heat due to qi vacuity

Example: *Huang Qi* (Radix Astragali Membranacei) + *Ren Shen* (Radix Panacis Ginseng)

Sweet + cold = Nourishing yin, moistening dryness, clearing heat

Example: *Mai Men Dong* (Tuber Ophiopogonis Japonici) + *Tian Men Dong* (Tuber Asparagi Cochinensis)

Sour + sweet = engendering yin

Example: *Bai Shao* (Radix Albus Paeoniae Lactiflorae) + *Zhi Gan Cao* (mix-fried Radix Glycyrrhizae)

Sour + sweet = relieving spasms & contractions

Example: *Bai Shao* (Radix Albus Paeoniae Lactiflorae) + *Zhi Gan Cao* (mix-fried Radix Glycyrrhizae)

Salty + cold = calming the liver & downbearing yang

Example: *Mu Li* (Conchae Ostreae) + *Shi Jue Ming* (Concha Haliotidis)

2
The Combinations

Bai He (Bulbus Lilii) & Zhi Mu (Rhizoma Anemarrhenae Aspheloidis)

Individual properties:	
Bai He	**Zhi Mu**
Nourishes heart yin and quiets the spirit Clears & moistens the lungs, stops coughing Sweet & cold but moistens without being slimy Tends to supplement Usual dosage: 10-30g	Clears heat and drains fire Enriches yin and moistens dryness Bitter & cold but drains fire without drying Tends to drain Usual dosage: 6-10g

Properties when combined:

One moistens, while the other clears.
One supplements, while the other drains.
When these two medicinals are combined
together, they moisten the lungs and clear heat,
nourish the heart and quiet the spirit.

Major indications of the combination:

1. Vexation and agitation, insomnia, vertigo,
thirst related to a warm disease which has
damaged yin or due to yin vacuity with vacuity
heat (1) (2)
2. Dry cough, vexation and agitation after a warm
disease (2)
3. Lily disease (3)

Notes:

(1) For these indications, this combination is
found in *Bai He Zhi Mu Tang* (Lily &
Anemarrhena Decoction).

(2) If dry cough is predominant, honey mix-fried
Bai He should be prescribed. If vexation and
agitation or insomnia is predominant, uncooked

Bai He should be prescribed. If thirst is
predominant, bran stir-fried *Zhi Mu* or honey
mix-fried *Zhi Mu* should be prescribed. If dry
cough is predominant, stir-fried till scorched *Zhi
Mu* should be prescribed.

(3) Lily disease is a form of mental depression
characterized by depressed emotions, anxiety,
taciturnity, a desire to sleep without being able to,
a desire to walk without being able to, a desire to
eat without being able to, a subjective feeling of
cold or hot, etc. This affection follows either a
warm disease, in which case it is of recent and
sudden onset, or emotional problems which have
damaged heart yin, in which case it is enduring
and progressive in nature. This disease bears the
name of the major plant which treats it, *Bai He*
(Bulbus Lilii).

Comment:

(a) *Bai He* is effective for the treatment of
numerous psychological or cardiac imbalances
related to heart yin vacuity, such as palpitations,
deep cardiac pain with a feeling of emptiness in
the cardiac area, insomnia, profuse dreams,
vexation and agitation, and neurasthenia.

Bai Ji (Rhizoma Bletillae Striatae) & *San Qi* (Radix Pseudoginseng)

Individual properties:	
Bai Ji	**San Qi**
Stops bleeding by astringing Disperses swelling, promotes granulation and engenders muscles (*i.e.*, flesh) Mainly treats bleeding from the lungs & stomach Usual dosage: 3-10g	Stops bleeding, quickens the blood, dispels stasis Disperses swelling Stops pain Treats all kinds of bleeding Usual dosage: 3-10g

Properties when combined:

One is fixed, while the other one is traveling.
One is astringing; the other is draining.
When these two medicinals are combined together, they act to mutually reinforce one another.

They effectively dispel stasis, stop bleeding, and engender muscle (*i.e.*, flesh) without producing blood stasis.

Major indications of the combination:

1. Hemoptysis (1)
2. Hematemesis (1)
3. Bleeding caused by trauma (2)

Notes:

(1) In clinical practice, it is the powder from these two medicinals that is used, 3-6g of each, 2-3 times per day. This mixture is very effective. Most bleeding can be stopped within two days. For gastric hemorrhages, it is advised to mix this powder with cool water in order to increase its vasoconstricting mechanism within the stomach. This helps stop the bleeding.

(2) For this purpose, apply this powder externally to the locally affected area.

Bai Ji Li (Fructus Tribuli Terrestris) & *Sha Yuan Zi* (Semen Astragali Complanati)

Individual properties:	
Bai Ji Li (a.k.a. Ji Li)	**Sha Yuan Zi (a.k.a. Sha Ji Li)**
Acrid, bitter, upbearing, dispersing Key tropism: the liver Calms the liver and resolves depression Dispels wind heat from liver channel and brightens the eyes Mainly treats repletion Usual dosage: 6-10g	Sweet, mild, supplementing, astringing Key tropism: the kidneys Supplements the kidneys and secures the essence Nourishes the liver and brightens the eyes Evenly supplements (*i.e.*, harmoniously supplements yin & yang) Mainly treats vacuity Usual dosage: 6-10g

Properties when combined:

One upbears; the other downbears.
One is channeled towards the liver; the other is channeled towards the kidneys.
When these two medicinals are combined, they regulate upbearing and downbearing and the kidneys and liver. They course the liver and rectify the qi, resolve depression and calm the liver. And they supplement harmoniously the liver and kidneys. This means that they enrich the kidneys and secure the essence, nourish the liver and brighten the eyes.

Major indications of the combination:

1. Vertigo, unclear vision due to liver and kidney vacuity (1)

2. Lumbar pain, seminal emission, premature ejaculation, frequent urination due to kidney vacuity (2)

3. Abnormal vaginal discharge due to kidney vacuity

Notes:

(1) For these indications, salt mix-fried *Bai Ji Li* should be prescribed. This preparation alleviates the draining and dispersing characteristics of *Bai Ji Li* and reinforces its supplementing aspect. This then should be combined with uncooked *Sha Yuan Zi.*

(2) For these indications, salt mix-fried *Sha Yuan Zi* or stir-fried *Sha Yuan Zi* should be prescribed.

Bai Qian (Radix Cynanchi Stautonii) & *Qian Hu* (Radix Peucedani)

Individual properties:	
Bai Qian	***Qian Hu***
Drains the lungs Downbears the qi Disperses phlegm[1] Treats cough and asthma due to an accumulation of phlegm with counterflow of lung qi Usual dosage: 6-10g	Dispels wind and diffuses the lung qi Downbears the qi Disperses phlegm Treats cough due to wind heat blocking the lung qi and causing qi counterflow Usual dosage: 6-10g

Properties when combined:

One downbears; the other diffuses. (1)
When these two medicinals are combined together, they mutually reinforce each other in order to disperse phlegm. In addition, they complement each other to downbear and diffuse the lung qi in order to effectively treat cough.

Major indications of the combination:
•

Cough with abundant phlegm or phlegm which is difficult to expectorate, itchy throat, chest

oppression due to blockage of the lung qi and lung qi counterflow. (2)

Notes:

(1) The lungs' function is to diffuse and to downbear. If external evils block the lung qi, this function of diffusing is disturbed. It is *Qian Hu* in particular which treats this disease mechanism. If the function of downbearing is disturbed (by external evils or an accumulation of phlegm), qi stagnates and reverses its flow. It is *Bai Qian* which particularly treats this disease mechanism.

---

[1]   *Xiao tan*, dispersing phlegm, is close to the Western idea of expectorating phlegm. It is different from *hua tan*, transforming phlegm which is a metabolic transformation.

(2) In case of cough caused by wind cold or wind heat, uncooked *Bai Qian* and uncooked *Qian Hu* should be prescribed. In case of cough caused by an accumulation of phlegm in the lungs, stir-fried till scorched *Bai Qian* and stir-fried till scorched *Qian Hu* should be prescribed. In case of chronic cough, dryness in lungs, or if the patient is old, use honey mix-fried *Bai Qian* and honey mix-fried *Qian Hu* in order to moisten the lungs.

Comments:

(a) *Bai Qian* is a medicinal substance with a wide spectrum of use which can be used in the treatment of almost every type of cough. (See (c) below.) This is why it is traditionally called "the essential medicinal of the lungs."

(b) Because the combination of *Bai Qian* and *Qian Hu* is complementary and very effective, these two medicinals are often combined in prescriptions treating cough and asthma and form a couple called *Er Qian*, the two *Qian*. This combination can be used in the treatment of numerous respiratory diseases: chronic bronchitis, dyspnea, asthma, whooping cough, cough associated with a cold, etc.

(c) *Bai Qian*, being neutral in nature, can be used in coughs due to either heat or cold. *Qian Hu*, slightly cold in nature, is used particularly for coughs due to wind heat, lung heat, or phlegm heat.

Bai Shao (Radix Albus Paeoniae Lactiflorae) & *Chai Hu* (Radix Bupleuri)

Individual properties:	
Bai Shao	***Chai Hu***
Acrid, cold, astringent	Acrid, sightly cold, dissipating
Nourishes the blood and constrains yin	Drains the liver and resolves depression
Harmonizes the constructive	Harmonizes the *shao yang*
Calms & emolliates the liver	Harmonizes the liver & spleen
Relieves tension[2]	Abates heat
Stops pain	Upbears clear yang
Usual dosage: 10-15g	Usual dosage: 5-15g

Properties when combined:

One is sour, while the other is acrid.
One is astringent; the other is dissipating.
These two are both directed toward the liver channel. When these two medicinals are combined together, they drain the liver without damaging liver yin, nourish the liver without causing liver depression qi stagnation, regulate the spleen and stop pain effectively. They also harmonize the exterior and the interior. Further, together, they constrain yin while upbearing yang.

Major indications of the combination:

1. Liver depression qi stagnation causing disharmony between the qi and blood (1)
2. Vertigo, unclear vision, chest and lateral costal oppression, pain, and distention due to liver depression qi stagnation or to disharmony between the exterior and interior (1) (2)
3. Menstrual irregularities, dysmenorrhea, breast distention, low-grade fever during the menses, premenstrual syndrome, and fibrocystic breasts, all caused by liver depression qi stagnation or

---

[2] *Jie ji*, to relieve or relax tension, is a treatment principle which can be applied to either physical tension, such as cramps, or mental-emotional tension.

disharmony between the liver and spleen (1) (3)

Notes:

(1) When pain is predominant, vinegar mix-fried *Chai Hu* is used advantageously. In case of liver-spleen disharmony, stir-fried *Chai Hu* should be prescribed. In case of vertigo, uncooked *Bai Shao* should be prescribed. In case of liver-spleen disharmony causing diarrhea, stir-fried till yellow *Bai Shao* should be prescribed. In case of gynecological problems, wine mix-fried *Bai Shao* should be prescribed. In case of chest or lateral costal pain, abdominal pain, or pain in the stomach area, wine mix-fried *Bao Shao* should be prescribed.

(2) For these indications, this combination is incorporated in *Chai Hu Shu Gan San* (Bupleurum Course the Liver Powder).

(3) For these indications, this combination is incorporated in *Xiao Yao San* (Rambling Powder).

Comments:

(a) This combination is effective for the treatment of liver and digestive problems caused by liver depression qi stagnation or to liver-spleen or liver-stomach disharmony, such as subacute or chronic hepatitis, hepatomegaly, cholecystitis, gallstones, enteritis, and colitis.

(b) *Chai Hu* is a messenger medicinal which guides the action of other medicinal substances towards the liver and gallbladder channels, towards the upper part of the body (*i.e.*, the head and face), along the liver channel pathway (internally) and the gallbladder channel pathway (externally), and towards the lateral costal region.

(c) *Chai Hu* in high dosage (10-18g) resolves the exterior, abates heat, and harmonizes the *shao yang*. In small dosage (2-4g), it upbears yang qi. In an average dosage (6-8g), it courses the liver, rectifies the qi, and resolves depression.

(d) *Chai Hu* originating from the southern provinces (Sichuan, Hubei, and Jiangsu) is called *Nan Chai Hu* (southern Bupleurum). It is superior for coursing the liver and resolving depression, as in *Chai Hu Shu Gan San* (Bupleurum Course the Liver Decoction), *Xiao Yao San* (Rambling Powder), and *Si Ni San* (Four Counterflows Powder). *Chai Hu* originating from the northern provinces (Liaoning, Gansu, Hebei, and Henan) is called *Bei Chai Hu* (northern Bupleurum). It is superior for harmonizing the *shao yang*, draining wind heat, and clearing heat, as in *Chai Hu Ge Gen Jie Ji Tang* (Bupleurum & Pueraria Resolve the Muscles Decoction), *Da Chai Hu Tang* (Major Bupleurum Decoction), and *Xiao Chai Hu Tang* (Minor Bupleurum Decoction).

Bai Shao (Radix Albus Paeoniae Lactiflorae) & Chi Shao (Radix Rubrus Paeoniae Lactiflorae)

Individual properties:	
Bai Shao	Chi Shao
Nourishes the blood and constrains yin Emolliates the liver and stops pain Nourishes liver yin (blood) Treats diseases of liver qi counterflowing upward caused by liver blood (yin) vacuity Supplements & constrains and does not drain Usual dosage: 6-10g	Clears heat and cools the blood Quickens the blood and dispels stasis Drains liver fire Treats disease of heat in the blood or blood stasis Drains and does not supplement Usual dosage: 6-10g

Properties when combined:

One constrains; the other drains.
One supplements; the other drains.
When these two medicinals are combined together, they nourish the blood, constrain yin, and cool the blood without engendering blood stasis. Further, together, they drain and nourish the liver and stop pain.

Major indications of the combination:

1. Persistent low-grade fever due to heat in blood (1)
2. Dry mouth and tongue, eyes red and painful due to insufficiency of fluids or yin caused by residual heat (1)
3. Lateral costal and chest pain, abdominal pain and conglomerations due to blood stasis or liver depression qi stagnation (2)
4. Menstrual irregularities or amenorrhea caused by blood stasis, blood vacuity, and /or liver depression qi stagnation (2)

Notes:

(1) For these indications, uncooked Bai Shao and uncooked Chi Shao should be prescribed, and thiscouple should be reinforced with uncooked Di Huang (Radix Rehmanniae), Di Gu Pi (Cortex Radicis Lycii Chinensis), and Mu Dan Pi (Cortex Radicis Moutan).

(2) For these indications, wine mix-fried Bai Shao and wine mix-fried Chi Shao should be prescribed and reinforced with Xiang Fu (Rhizoma Cyperi Rotundi) and Dang Gui (Radix Angelica Sinensis).

Comments:

(a) Cold's nature is to contract the blood vessels and congeal the blood. This is why Chi Shao, which quickens the blood and drains stasis, is used when a lot of cooling the blood medicinals are being prescribed, thus preventing blood stasis.

(b) Chi Shao treats hepatitis A and B (it regulates gamma GT and transaminases) due to liver fire or liver blood stasis. However, most hepatitis and especially enduring cases are accompanied by blood stasis. It is, therefore, advantageous to prescribe Chi Shao (10-30g/day depending on the severity of the stasis) on a routine basis in this disease.

Bai Shao (Radix Albus Paeoniae Lactiflorae) & Gan Cao (Radix Glycyrrhizae)

Individual properties:	
Bai Shao	**Gan Cao**
Nourishes the blood and constrains yin Soothes the liver and calms the liver Relieves tension and stops pain Because it is sour, *Bai Shao* is focused on the liver and treats wood. Method of preparation: wine mix-fried Usual dosage: 10-15g (up to 60g)	Supplements the central qi Harmonizes other medicinals Soothes the sinews and stops pain Because it is sweet, *Gan Cao* is focused on the spleen and treats earth. Method of preparation: honey mix-fried Usual dosage: 6-10g

Properties when combined:

One is sour, while the other is sweet.
One focuses on the liver; the other on the spleen.
When these two medicinals are combined together, sweet and sour engender yin. (1) Together, they effectively calm the liver and fortify the spleen, supplement the qi and blood, and harmonize the liver and spleen. In addition, they soothe the sinews and stop pain.

Major indications of the combination:

1. Weakness in the lower limbs and spasms and pain in the limbs due to disharmony between the qi and the blood which causes inadequate nourishment of the sinews and vessels (2)
2. Abdominal pain due to liver-spleen disharmony (2)
3. Headaches due to blood vacuity (3)

Notes:

(1) The expressions, to transform yin, and, to transform yang, describe the result obtained by the combination of different flavors. The sour and sweet flavors engender yin, while the acrid and sweet engender yang. Therefore, there is no direct influx of yin substance or yang qi. Rather, this engenderment of yin and yang is due to these medicinals' indirect nutritional contribution. Hence they are not slimy nor hard to digest and do not cause accumulation. Instead, yin and yang are transformed via the transformative functions of the spleen.

(2) For these indications, this combination is present in *Shao Yao Gan Cao Tang* (Peony & Licorice Decoction). If the disorder is accompanied by cold signs, one can use wine mix-fried *Bai Shao* and mix-fried *Gan Cao*. If the disorder is accompanied by heat signs, one can use uncooked *Bai Shao* (or *Chi Shao*) and uncooked *Gan Cao*.

(3) For this indication, one can add *He Shou Wu* (Radix Polygoni Multiflori), *Bai Ji Li* (Fructus Tribuli Terrestris), and *Jiang Can* (Bombyx Batryticatus) which favorably reinforce this combination.

Comments:

(a) This combination is very effective for numerous problems accompanied by spasms and pain, such as gastritis or colitis, spasm of the gastrocnemius muscle in the leg, contraction of the limbs, tendinitis, lateral costal pain, and hiccup or stubborn vomiting caused by spasm of the diaphragm.

(b) In case of edema, oliguria, anuria, or hypertension, the dosage of *Gan Cao* or mix-fried *Gan Cao* must be moderate (3-6g) and its administration should be of short duration. This is because this medicinal encourages sodium retention. In other cases, for prolonged administration, a dosage of 10g per day should not be exceeded.

(c) *Gan Cao* is incompatible with pork meat, seaweed (particularly *Hai Zao* [Herba Sargassii]), and Chinese cabbage (*Brassica Chinensis* or *Brassica Pekinensis*).

Bai Shao (Radix Albus Paeoniae Lactiflorae) & *Gui Zhi* (Ramulus Cinnamomi Cassiae)

Individual properties:	
Bai Shao	*Gui Zhi*
Bitter, sour, cold Harmonizes the constructive qi Constrains & protects yin Nourishes the blood and constrains yin without attracting nor blocking evils in the interior Tropism: the yin division Relieves tension and stops pain Nourishes stomach yin Usual dosage: 6-10g	Acrid, sweet, warm Harmonizes the constructive qi Promotes perspiration Promotes perspiration and resolves the exterior without damaging yin Tropism: the blood division Warms the channels and quickens the network vessels Supplements spleen yang Usual dosage: 6-10g

Properties when combined:

One is cool and sour, while the other is warm and acrid.
One is astringent, while the other is scattering.
One assists yin; the other assists yang.
One releases; the other moves.
One is for yin; the other is for yang.
When these two medicinals are combined together, they harmonize yin and yang, the qi and blood, and the constructive and defensive. Together, they drain without damaging yin, while they constrain yin without retaining evils. In addition, they harmonize the vessels, relieve tension, and stop pain, as well as support stomach yin and spleen yang, while regulating the spleen and stomach.

Major indications of the combination:

1. Common cold with fever, shivers, slight perspiration, no thirst, headache, thin, white tongue fur, and a floating, moderate pulse or, in other words, a wind cold exterior pattern with disharmony between the constructive and defensive (1) (4)
2. Spontaneous perspiration and/or night sweats accompanied by fear of wind and cold, a cold feeling in the low back, and frequent catching of colds due to disharmony between the constructive and defensive (1) (5)
3. Chest and cardiac area pain due to heart yang vacuity and disharmony between the qi and blood (6)
4. Abdominal pain with spasms and cramps due to vacuity cold and disharmony between the qi and blood (2) (7)
5. Pain and/or numbness of the limbs due to disharmony between the qi and blood (3) (6)
6. Vomiting and weakness during pregnancy accompanied by fear of cold, lack of appetite, nausea, and a weak pulse in the cubit position due to disharmony of the spleen and stomach and constructive and defensive (1) (6)
7. Weakness in the elderly, during convalescence, postpartum, and post-operatively with fatigue and lack of strength, fear of wind, and slight perspiration due to disharmony between the constructive and defensive (1) (5)

Notes:

(1) For this indication, this combination is present in *Gui Zhi Tang* (Cinnamon Twig Decoction). In

this case, the dosage of *Gui Zhi* and *Bai Shao* should be equal. For indications No.1 (but not for #2, 6, or 7), the patient should be advised that, 10 minutes after taking the decoction, they should eat a very hot rice soup and stay well covered in bed in order to promote perspiration. In any case, when *Gui Zhi Tang* is used, one must avoid eating raw, cold, or greasy foods as well as taking alcohol and meat.

(2) For this indication, this combination is present in *Xiao Jian Zhong Tang* (Minor Fortify the Center Decoction). In this case, the dosage of *Bai Shao* should be twice as much as the dosage of *Gui Zhi*.

(3) For this indication, *Gui Zhi* is used at a higher dosage: 15-30g. In case of very cold limbs, *Fu Zi* (Radix Lateralis Praeparatus Aconitii Carmichaeli) can be added, as in *Gui Zhi Fu Zi Tang* (Cinnamon Twig & Aconite Decoction).

(4) For these indications, uncooked *Gui Zhi* and uncooked *Bai Shao* should be prescribed.

(5) For these indications, stir-fried *Gui Zhi* and uncooked *Bai Shao* should be prescribed.

(6) For these indications, stir-fried *Gui Zhi* and wine mix-fried *Bai Shao* should be prescribed.

(7) For these indications, honey mix-fried *Gui Zhi* and wine mix-fried *Bai Shao* should be prescribed.

Comments:

(a) Usually, the defensive and constructive qi regulate and balance each other. The defensive qi is associated with yang and controls the exterior, while the constructive qi is associated with yin and controls the interior. Together, they secure the exterior and interior and participate in the yin-yang balance of the organism. In case of exterior attack, if the defensive qi (which may be weak prior to the attack) focuses all its power towards the exterior in order to fight the evil qi, the result may be a disharmony between the defensive and constructive. In that case, the defensive no longer can requisition sufficient fluids from the constructive necessary to effectively expel the evils. Simultaneously, the defensive qi is involved in fighting the evils in the exterior. Therefore, it is no longer available to maintain and support the constructive qi in the interior. This causes a rupture in the exchange between these two qi, causing an imbalance between yin and yang. The constructive qi is no longer anchored in the interior and thus becomes unstable and no longer controls fluids (yin). These then escape towards the exterior. The result is spontaneous perspiration but which is not sufficient to expel the exterior evils.

This is the situation for which this combination is indicated *vis a vis* a wind cold exterior pattern with disharmony of the defensive and constructive. The therapeutic strategy consists of keeping those fluids which are escaping spontaneously to the exterior because of disharmony of the defensive and constructive in the interior at the same time as triggering a strong, *voluntary* perspiration in order to expel the evil qi. Thus, *Gui Zhi* reinforces the defensive qi and supports yang qi. *Bai Shao* reinforces the constructive qi and constrains yin. Together, they harmonize the constructive and defensive, re-establish interaction between these two qi, and reinstate the yin-yang balance in order to stop spontaneous perspiration. In this way, efficient perspiration is achieved and the evils are expelled.

(b) *Gui Zhi Jian* or *Gui Zhi Shao* (Extremitas Ramuli Cinnamomi Cassiae) are the fine twigs of Cinnamon. They are known for their powerful qi and are very fragrant. They are more powerful for scattering wind cold, warming and opening the channels and vessels, and quickening the blood.

Bai Zhu (Rhizoma Atractylodis Macrocephalae) & *Fu Ling* (Sclerotium Poriae Cocos)

Individual properties:	
Bai Zhu	**Fu Ling**
Sweet, warm, supplementing Strongly supplements the spleen & qi (1) Dries dampness (1) Disinhibits water (1) Superior in supplementing the spleen and drying dampness Usual dosage: 10-15g	Sweet, bland, disinhibits urination Mildly supplements the spleen & middle burner Percolates dampness Disinhibits water Superior for percolating dampness and disinhibiting urination without injuring the correct qi Usual dosage: 10-15g

Properties when combined:

One supplements, while the other percolates. One is drying, the other disinhibits urination. When these two medicinals are combined together, they reinforce each other. Together, they effectively supplement the spleen and dry dampness, percolate dampness and disinhibit urination.

Major indications of the combination:

1. Edema due to accumulation of dampness in turn caused by spleen vacuity (3)
2. Fatigue, weakness in limbs, lack of appetite, loose stools or diarrhea caused by spleen vacuity with accumulation of dampness (4)
3. Vertigo, blurred vision, and/or heart palpitations due to phlegm dampness (5)
4. Chronic cough due to phlegm dampness and spleen vacuity (6)

Notes:

(1) To fortify the spleen and supplement the qi, bran stir-fried *Bai Zhu* is prescribed. To dry dampness and disinhibit urination, uncooked *Bai Zhu* is prescribed.

(2) Percolating dampness is a therapeutic method using medicinal substances with a bland taste, for example, *Yi Yi Ren* (Semen Coicis Lachryma-jobi), *Fu Ling* (Sclerotium Poriae Cocos), *Ze Xie* (Rhizoma Alismatis), and *Zhu Ling* (Sclerotium Polypori Umbellati) in order to gradually eliminate dampness in the treatment of oliguria, edema, phlegm dampness, diarrhea, etc.

(3) For this indication, this combination is used in *Bai Zhu San* (Atractylodes Powder).

(4) For these indications, this combination is used in *Shen Ling Bai Zhu San* (Ginseng, Poria & Atractylodes Powder).

(5) For these indications, this combination is used in *Ling Gui Zhu Gan Tang* (Poriae, Cinnamon, Atractylodes & Licorice Decoction).

(6) For these indications, this combination is used in *Liu Jun Zi Tang* (Six Gentlemen Decoction).

Comments:

(a) *Bai Zhu* is incompatible with black carp, peach, plum, coriander, and Chinese cabbage (*Brassica Chinensis* or *Brassica Pekinensis*). *Fu Ling* is incompatible with tea, vinegar, and all very sour foods.

(b) *Fu Ling* is a generic term for the mushroom which parasitizes the roots of *Pinus densiflora* and *Pinus massoniana*. It is subdivided into the following particular medicinals:

i. *Fu Ling Pi* (Cortex Sclerotii Poriae Cocos)

This consists of the blackish bark of the mushroom. It disinhibits urination without affecting the qi. It disperses swelling and treats edema and oliguria caused by a severe accumulation of dampness in turn due to spleen vacuity. Its action is draining and slightly supplementing. Usual dosage: 15-30g

ii. *Chi Fu Ling* or *Chi Ling* (Sclerotium Rubrum Poriae Cocos)

This consists of the pinkish, most external flesh located just under the blackish bark. It drains heat and disinhibits urination, while it treats strangury, oliguria, and red or dark-colored urine due to damp heat. Its action is draining. Usual dosage: 5-15g

iii. *Fu Ling*, *Bai Fu Ling*, or *Yun Fu Ling* (Sclerotium Album Poriae Cocos)

This consists of the whitish flesh which is the largest constituent of the mushroom. It disinhibits urination, supplements the spleen, and quiets the spirit. It treats edema, oliguria, and phlegm due to spleen vacuity, nausea and vomiting due to stagnation of dampness in the middle burner, and loss of appetite and diarrhea due to spleen vacuity. Its action is supplementing and moderately draining without affecting the qi. Usual dosage: 5-15g

iv. *Fu Shen* (Sclerotium Pararadicis Poriae Cocos)

This consists of the flesh surrounding the parasitized root. It calms the heart and quiets the spirit and treats insomnia, disturbed sleep, heart palpitations, and loss of memory. Its action of quieting the spirit is stronger than that of *Bai Fu Ling*. When *Fu Shen* is prepared with *Zhu Sha* (Cinnabar), this strengthens its calming effect even more. Usual dosage: 5-15g

v. *Fu Shen Xin* (Centrum Sclerotii Pararadicis Poriae Cocos)

This consists of the parasitized root of the pine which is at the heart of the mushroom. It calms the liver, tranquilizes the heart and quiets the spirit, and drains wind and dampness. It treats insomnia, cardiac pain, and spasms of the sinews. Its action of quieting the spirit is superior to either *Bai Fu Ling* or *Fu Shen*. Usual dosage: 5-10g

Bai Zhu (Rhizoma Atractylodis Macrocephalae) & *Huang Qin* (Radix Scutellariae Baicalensis)

Individual properties:	
Bai Zhu	**Huang Qin**
Supplements the qi & the middle burner Fortifies the spleen to maintain the blood within its vessels Dries cold dampness Quiets & secures the fetus Usual dosage: 10-15g	Clears heat Drains lung, liver, gallbladder & large intestine fire Clears and eliminates damp heat Clears heat and quiets the fetus Usual dosage: 6-12g

Properties when combined:

One is warm, while the other is cold.
One supplements; the other drains.

The two are main medicinals for quieting the fetus.
When these two medicinals are combined together, they clear heat stirring the fetus, dry dampness, and fortify the spleen to contain the

blood and the fetus. Thus, as a combination they effectively quiet the fetus.

Major indications of the combination:

1. Uterine bleeding during pregnancy, threatened miscarriage, nausea and vomiting during pregnancy caused by heat or damp heat associated with spleen vacuity which is incapable of containing the blood within its vessels (1) (2)

Notes:

(1) For these indications, this combination is used in *Bai Zhu San* (Atractylodes Powder [II]). If the patient also suffers from qi stagnation, add *Sha Ren* (Fructus Amomi) and *Zi Su Geng* (Caulis Perillae Frutescentis). If she suffers from blood vacuity, add *Dang Gui* (Radix Angelicae Sinensis) and *Bai Shao* (Radix Albus Paeoniae Lactiflorae). If she suffers from kidney vacuity, add *Xu Duan* (Radix Dipsaci) and *Sang Ji Sheng* (Ramulus Loranthi Seu Visci). If she suffers from qi vacuity, add *Ren Shen* (Radix Panacis Ginseng) and *Huang Qi* (Radix Astragali Membranacei). If she suffers from heat, add *Nan Gua Di* (Pediculus Cucurbitae) and *Zhu Ma Gen* (Radix Boehmeriae). If she suffers from

metrorrhagia, add *E Jiao* (Gelatinum Corii Asini), *Han Lian Cao* (Herba Ecliptae Prostratae), and *Xian He Cao* (Herba Agrimoniae Pilosae). If she suffers from nausea and vomiting, add *Huang Lian* (Rhizoma Coptidis Chinensis) and *Zi Su Ye* (Folium Perillae Frutescentis).

(2) For these indications, bran stir-fried *Bai Zhu* and stir-fried till scorched *Huang Qin* should be prescribed.

Comments:

(a) Women by nature are yin. During pregnancy, yang becomes stronger and easily produces heat. This is because the creation of the fetus is a warm transformation and also because the child's qi is added to the mothers. As a result, clinically, it is frequent to see a restlessly stirring fetus due to qi stagnation, qi and/or blood vacuity, or kidney vacuity which is associated with heat. That is the reason why *Huang Qin* can almost always be prescribed for this type of problem.

(b) *Bai Zhu* is incompatible with black carp, peach, plum, coriander, and Chinese cabbage (*Brassica Chinensis* or *Brassica Pekinensis*).

Bai Zhu (Rhizoma Atractylodis Macrocephalae) & *Zhi Shi* (Fructus Immaturus Citri Aurantii)

Individual properties:	
Bai Zhu	**Zhi Shi**
Sweet, warm, moderately supplementing	Acrid, warm, drastically draining
Fortifies the spleen and dries dampness	Breaks the qi (1)
Disperses swelling	Disperses accumulations & distention
Harmonizes the center	Disperses food stagnation and frees the flow of
Quiets the fetus	the stools
Fixed in nature	Traveling in nature
Usual dosage: 10-15g	Usual dosage: 5-10g

Properties when combined:

One supplements, while the other drains.
One is moderate, while the other is drastic.

One is fixed; the other is mobile.
When these two medicinals are combined together, they supplement without producing stagnation and drain without damaging the

correct qi. Together, they fortify the spleen, disperse food stagnation, and effectively eliminate accumulations and distention.

Major indications of the combination:

1. Accumulation of food, distention and fullness of the abdomen and epigastrium, and difficult bowel movements due to spleen qi vacuity and qi stagnation (2)
2. Splenomegaly and hepatomegaly due to qi vacuity and stagnation
3. Ptosis of the organs (stomach, uterus, and anus) due to central qi vacuity (3)

Notes:

(1) Breaking the qi is a therapeutic method aimed at treating severe qi stagnation with drastic medicinal substances, for example, *Zhi Shi* (Fructus Immaturus Citri Aurantii) or *Qing Pi* (Pericarpium Citri Reticulatae Viride).
(2) For these indications, this combination is used in *Zhi Zhu Wan* (Citrus & Atractylodes Pills). When the patient's main complaint is abdominal and epigastric distention due to qi vacuity and spleen vacuity with or without dampness, the dosage for *Bai Zhu* should be very high, as much

as 100g per day. In this case, *Bai Zhu* is generally used alone. *Dong Bai Zhu* (Atractylodes harvested in winter), instead of having a dry character like *Bai Zhu*, has a moistening one. It fortifies spleen yang and nourishes spleen yin, moistens the intestines and treats constipation. In this case, *Dong Bai Zhu* is simply washed and dried in the sun.

(3) For these indications, this combination is favorably reinforced by honey mix-fried *Huang Qi* (Radix Astragali Membranacei), stir-fried *Chai Hu* (Radix Bupleuri), and honey mix-fried *Sheng Ma* (Rhizoma Cimicifugae). *Zhi Shi* strongly moves and downbears the qi. However, in clinical practice, like *Zhi Ke* (Fructus Citri Aurantii), it very effectively treats prolapse of the anus caused by central qi fall. These two medicinals are particularly indicated in cases of prolapse of the anus in conjunction with constipation.

Comment:

(a) For all these indications, except as otherwise indicated, it is recommended to prescribe bran stir-fried *Bai Zhu* and stir-fried *Zhi Shi*.

Bai Zi Ren (Semen Biotae Orientalis) & *Suan Zao Ren* (Semen Zizyphi Spinosae)

Individual properties:	
Bai Zi Ren	**Suan Zao Ren**
Supplements the heart qi & blood Quiets the *hun, po* & *shen* Superior for supplementing the heart Treats heart palpitations caused by heart vacuity Boosts the intelligence Moistens the intestines Usual dosage: 10-15g	Nourishes heart yin & blood Quiets the *hun* & *shen* Superior for supplementing the liver & gallbladder Treats heart palpitations due to gallbladder vacuity Nourishes liver blood Stops perspiration by astringing Usual dosage: 10-15g

Properties when combined:

Together, they reinforce each other's actions. They effectively nourish both the liver and heart and tranquilize the heart and quiet the spirit.

Major indications of the combination:

1. Heart palpitations, profuse dreams, and insomnia due to heart blood (and qi) vacuity (1)
2. Constipation with dry stools due to blood vacuity or intestinal fluid insufficiency

Notes:

(1) For these indications, this combination is used in *Tian Wang Bu Xin Dan* (Heavenly Emperor Supplement the Heart Elixir). For these indications, defatted *Bai Zi Ren* and stir-fried *Suan Zao Ren* should be prescribed.

(2) For these indications, uncooked *Bai Zi Ren* should be prescribed.

Ban Lan Gen (Radix Isatidis Seu Baphicacanthi) & *Shan Dou Gen* (Radix Sophorae Subprostratae)

Individual properties:	
Ban Lan Gen	*Shan Dou Gen*
Bitter, cold Clears heat and resolves toxins Disinhibits the throat Tends to treat heat toxins in the blood division Usual dosage: 10-15g	Very bitter, very cold Clears heat and resolves toxins Disperses swelling and stops pain Disinhibits the throat Tends to treat fire toxins rising upward Usual dosage: 6-12g

Properties when combined:

When these two medicinals are combined together, they reinforce each other. As a combination, they clear heat, resolve toxins, and strongly disinhibit the throat.

Major indications of the combination:

1. Painful, red, and swollen throat due to replete heat (1)
2. Toothache and painful, swollen gums due to replete heat
3. Oral ulcers due to replete heat

Notes:

(1) For this indication, this combination is usually sufficient to treat severe throat inflammations (including strep throat, tonsillitis, pharyngitis, laryngitis, etc.) due to heat toxins or replete heat. However, when this combination needs further reinforcement, *She Gan* (Rhizoma Belamcandae), *Jin Yin Hua* (Flos Lonicerae Japonicae), *Lian Qiao* (Fructus Forsythiae Suspensae), *Xuan Shen* (Radix Scrophulariae Ningpoensis), and *Gan Cao* (Radix Glycyrrhizae) may also be prescribed. *Shan Dou Gen* is the most efficient Chinese medicinal to treat throat inflammations due to heat toxins or replete heat.

Ban Lan Gen (Radix Isatidis Seu Baphicacanthi) & Xuan Shen (Radix Scrophulariae Ningpoensis)

Individual properties:	
Ban Lan Gen	**Xuan Shen**
Bitter, cold Clears heat and resolves toxins Cools the blood Disinhibits the throat and disperses swelling Usual dosage: 10-15g	Sweet, bitter, cold Nourishes yin, drains fire (and floating fire), and resolves toxins Cools the blood Disinhibits the throat Usual dosage: 10-15g

Properties when combined:

One clears, while the other nourishes.
One clears heat, the other downbears fire.
When these two medicinals are combined together, they clear heat and resolves\ toxins, cool the blood and nourish yin, downbear fire and disinhibit the throat, disperse swelling and stop pain.

Major indications of the combination:

1. Painful, red, swollen throat with dry, red tongue, and a fine, rapid pulse due to yin vacuity generating a vacuity fire or replete fire which damages yin (1)

Note:

(1) If heat toxins are present, this combination can be advantageously reinforced with *Shan Dou* *Gen* (Radix Sophorae Subprostratae) and *Gan Cao* (Radix Glycyrrhizae). If there is vacuity fire, this combination can be advantageously reinforced by *Mai Men Dong* (Tuber Ophiopogonis Japonici) and uncooked *Di Huang* (Radix Rehmanniae). For these indications, *Ban Lan Gen* can easily be replaced by *Da Qing Ye* (Folium Isatidis) without changing the efficiency of the combination.

Comment:

(a) In ancient China, nothing and nobody could bear the emperor's name. This is called name taboo by sinologists. During the reign of the second Emperor of the Qing dynasty, Kang Xi, also called Xuan Ye, *Xuan Shen* was renamed *Yuan Shen*. This is why this synonym is commonly found in modern Chinese materia medica.

Ban Xia (Rhizoma Pinelliae Ternatae) & Chen Pi (Pericarpium Citri Reticulatae)

Individual properties:	
Ban Xia	**Chen Pi**
Dries dampness and transforms phlegm Scatters nodulation Downbears qi and stops vomiting Usual dosage: 6-10g	Rectifies the qi and moderately fortifies the spleen Dries dampness and transforms phlegm Harmonizes the stomach and stops vomiting Usual dosage: 6-10g

Properties when combined:

When these two medicinals are combined together, they mutually reinforce one another. Together, they fortify the spleen, rectify the qi, dry dampness, transform phlegm and stop vomiting.

Major indications of the combination:

1. Cough due to an accumulation of phlegm dampness (1)
2. Chest oppression, nausea, and vomiting due to stomach disharmony and phlegm damp stagnation (2)

Notes:

(1) For this indication, this combination is present in *Er Chen Tang* (Two Aged [Medicinals] Decoction). Some medicinals are stored and aged in order to reduce their secondary effects and reinforce their therapeutic action. The longer they are kept, the more efficient and the less secondary effects. Traditionally, six aged medicinals are discussed in the Chinese medical literature. *Ban Xia* and *Chen Pi* are among these medicinals and are the two aged ingredients in *Er Chen Tang*. They dry dampness without damaging yin and move the qi without damaging the correct qi. The four others are: *Zhi Ke* (Fructus Citri Aurantii), *Ma Huang* (Herba Ephedrae), *Wu Zhu Yu* (Fructus Evodiae Rutecarpae), and *Lang Du* (Radix Stellariae Chamaejasmi). For this indication, lime-processed *Ban Xia* and uncooked *Chen Pi* should be prescribed.

(2) For these indications, this combination is present in *Er Chen Tang* (Two Aged [Medicinals] Decoction). For these indications, ginger-processed *Ban Xia* and stir-fried *Chen Pi* should be prescribed.

Comments:

(a) To treat phlegm dampness, three essential therapeutic methods are used. The first one consists of making the phlegm already existing disappear by transforming and drying it or by evacuating it through expectoration. The second consists of moving the qi. If qi moves with fluidity, phlegm is expelled through expectoration and stagnant dampness, which is the origin of the production of phlegm, is moved and does not accumulate. Thus that dampness does not congeal into phlegm. This is based on the classical saying, "To treat phlegm, one must first treat the qi." According to Pang An-shi (1042-1099 CE):

> When treating phlegm, do not treat phlegm but treat the qi. When the qi flow is normalized, the fluids of the entire body will also follow the qi and be normalized.

The third method consists of supplementing the spleen. Phlegm dampness is often engendered by stagnant dampness in turn due to spleen vacuity. By fortifying the spleen, one promotes the transformation and transportation of water and grain and thus prevents accumulation of evil dampness and the engenderment of phlegm. It is interesting to note that *Chen Pi* includes the three essential functions necessary to eliminate phlegm dampness. It transforms phlegm, moves the qi, and fortifies the spleen. *Er Chen Tang* also contains these three therapeutic strategies to treat phlegm: to transform (*Ban Xia* & *Chen Pi*), to move (*Chen Pi*), to supplement (*Fu Ling* & *Zhi Gan Cao*). This is why this formula is the basis of many other formulas for various types of phlegm conditions, vacuity or repletion, cold or heat, external or internal.

(b) *Ban Xia* is incompatible with mutton and sheep blood eaten as a food and maltose (*Yi Tang*).

Ban Xia (Tuber Pinelliae Ternatae) & Huang Lian (Rhizoma Coptidis Chinensis)

Individual properties:	
Ban Xia	**Huang Lian**
Acrid, warm, drying, and frees the flow Transforms phlegm and dries dampness Downbears qi counterflow Frees the flow of and eliminates dampness accumulated in the middle burner Usual dosage: 6-10g	Bitter, cold, drying, draining Clears heat and dries dampness Clears the stomach, liver & heart Drains and eliminates heat accumulated in the middle burner Usual dosage: 6-10g

Properties when combined:

One is warm, while the other is cold.
One is acrid; the other is bitter.
One frees the flow; the other drains.
The acrid taste and warm nature favor the spleen.
Bitter and cool favors the stomach.
When these two medicinals are combined together, acrid and bitter, cool and warm harmonize upbearing and downbearing, yin and yang. Together, they clear heat and dry dampness, transform phlegm and stop vomiting.

Major indications of the combination:

1. Nausea, vomiting, chest and epigastric fullness and distention, thick, yellow phlegm, yellow, slimy tongue fur, and a wiry, slippery pulse due to damp heat, turbid phlegm, and/or mixed cold and heat causing stomach disharmony (1)

Notes:

(1) For these indications, this combination is used in *Huang Lian Tang* (Coptis Decoction). For these indications, ginger-processed *Ban Xia* and ginger mix-fried *Huang Lian* should be prescribed.

Comment:

(a) *Huang Lian* is incompatible with pork or cold water. *Ban Xia* is incompatible with mutton, sheep's blood and Maltose (*Yi Tang*).

Ban Xia (Rhizoma Pinelliae Ternatae) & Huang Qin (Radix Scutellariae Baicalensis)

Individual properties:	
Ban Xia	**Huang Qin**
Acrid, draining Fortifies the spleen and dries dampness Harmonizes the stomach and stops vomiting Scatters nodulation Downbears qi counterflow Usual dosage: 6-10g	Bitter, cold Clears heat and dries dampness Drains fire and resolves toxins Stops bleeding and quiets the fetus Usual dosage: 6-10g

Properties when combined:

One is warm, while the other is cold.
One is acrid and frees the flow; the other is bitter and drains.
When these two medicinals are combined together, they harmonize and re-establish the interaction between yin and yang. Together, they effectively clear heat and drain fire, harmonize the stomach and stop vomiting, and scatter nodulation.

Major indications of the combination:

1. Vomiting and nausea due to *shao yang* pattern (1)
2. Phlegm heat (2)
3. Lack of appetite, nausea, vomiting, and distention and sensation of fullness in the stomach, diaphragm, and chest caused by a pattern of mixed cold and heat (3)

Notes:

(1) For these indications, this combination is present in *Xiao Chai Hu Tang* (Minor Bupleurum Decoction). For these indications, one should prescribe ginger-processed *Ban Xia* and uncooked *Huang Qin*.

(2) For this indication, this combination is used in *Qing Qi Hua Tan Wan* (Clear the Qi & Transform Phlegm Pills). For this indication, one should prescribe lime-processed *Ban Xia* and wine mix-fried *Huang Qin*.

(3) For these indications, this combination is used in *Ban Xia Xie Xin Tang* (Pinelliae Drain the Heart Decoction). For these indications, one should prescribe ginger-processed *Ban Xia* and stir-fried till scorched *Huang Qin*, bran stir-fried *Huang Qin*, or ginger mix-fried *Huang Qin*.

Comment:

(a) The combination of *Ban Xia* & *Huang Qin* and *Chai Hu* & *Huang Qin* (see the combination below) in *Xiao Chai Hu Tang* (Minor Bupleurum Decoction) to resolve the *shao yang* division is well evidenced by clinical practice. In such cases, when *Huang Qin* is removed, the pain and distention of the chest and lateral costal regions disappear, but the alternating fever and chills persist. When *Ban Xia* is removed, the fever and chills disappear, but the pain and distention of the chest and lateral costal regions persist. When *Chai Hu* is used alone, the fever does not abate, but if *Huang Qin* is added, the fever recedes efficiently.

Ban Xia (Rhizoma Pinelliae Ternatae) & *Sheng Jiang* (Uncooked Rhizoma Zingiberis)

Individual properties:	
Ban Xia	***Sheng Jiang***
Transforms phlegm Downbears qi counterflow and stops vomiting Treats vomiting due to accumulation of phlegm in the stomach Usual dosage: 6-10g	Warms the center and stops vomiting Drains yin fluids accumulated in the center Treats vomiting caused by cold in the stomach Usual dosage: 6-10g

Properties when combined:

One downbears, while the other drains.
One dries; the other warms.
When these two medicinals are combined together, they transform phlegm and downbear counterflow, harmonize the stomach and stop vomiting.

Major indications of the combination:

1. Nausea, vomiting with no thirst, and slimy tongue fur due to phlegm dampness stagnating in the middle burner (1) (2)
2. Enduring cough with white, watery, and profuse phlegm (3)

Notes:

(1) For these indications, this combination is used in *Xiao Ban Xia Tang* (Minor Pinellia Decoction). For these indications, ginger-processed *Ban Xia* should be prescribed.

(2) *Sheng Jiang* is renowned for effectively treating vomiting. It can be used for all types of vomiting, even in the case of stomach heat, if it is combined with other medicinals related to the nature of the imbalance. It is traditionally said, "*Sheng Jiang* is a sagelike medicinal for vomiting." Another interesting application of *Sheng Jiang* is to use it with bitter medicinals when these would otherwise cause nausea. In that case, *Sheng Jiang* is directly integrated into the decoction or chewed immediately after swallowing the liquid. This often is sufficient "to calm the most stubborn patient."

(3) For these indications, this combination is present in *Er Chen Tang* (Two Aged [Medicinals] Decoction) and all its variations. For these indications, lime-processed *Ban Xia* should be prescribed.

Ban Xia (Rhizoma Pinelliae Ternatae) & *Shu Mi* (Semen Panici Miliacei)

Individual properties:	
Ban Xia	**Shu Mi**
Transforms phlegm Disperses food stagnation (1) Harmonizes the stomach Downbears counterflowing qi Usual dosage: 6-10g	Supplements the stomach qi Transforms phlegm Harmonizes the stomach Quiets the spirit Usual dosage: 12g

Properties when combined:

Together, these two medicinals transform phlegm, harmonize the stomach, and quiet the spirit.

Major indications of the combination:

1. Insomnia with heart palpitations, nausea, and cough with thin phlegm due to phlegm dampness accumulation in the middle burner causing stomach disharmony (2)

Notes:

(1) For this indication, it is worthwhile to use *Ban Xia Qu* (Pinellia Massa Medica Fermentata).

(2) For these indications, this combination is used in *Ban Xia Shu Mi Tang* (Pinellia & Millet Decoction).

Comment:

(a) *Ban Xia* and *Shu Mi* is the major combination and probably the best to treat insomnia due to stomach disharmony, *i.e.*, stagnant food preventing the defensive qi from entering the interior.

Ban Xia (Rhizoma Pinelliae Ternatae) & Zhu Ru (Caulis Bambusae In Taeniis)

Individual properties:	
Ban Xia	*Zhu Ru*
Downbears the qi and stops vomiting Dries dampness and transforms phlegm Warm, transforms phlegm dampness and cold phlegm rheum which is profuse and easy to expectorate Treats vomiting due to accumulation of phlegm dampness and stomach disharmony Usual dosage: 6-10g	Clears heat and stops vomiting Downbears the qi and eliminates phlegm Cool, eliminates thick and sticky phlegm heat Treats vomiting due to stomach heat and counterflow of stomach qi Usual dosage: 6-10g

Properties when combined:

One is warm, while the other is cool. When these two medicinals are combined together, they mutually reinforce each other. Together, they effectively dry dampness, clear heat, transform phlegm, harmonize the stomach, and stop vomiting.

Major indications of the combination:

1. Hiccup, nausea, and vomiting due to disharmony and counterflow of stomach qi (1)
2. Vertigo, agitation, and insomnia due to phlegm turbidity (2)3. Nausea and vomiting during pregnancy due to disharmony of the stomach, phlegm heat, or heat in the stomach (1) (3)

Notes:

(1) For these indications, ginger-processed *Ban Xia* and ginger mix-fried *Zhu Ru* should be prescribed.
(2) For these indications, lime-processed *Ban Xia* and ginger-processed *Zhu Ru* should be prescribed.
(3) To reinforce the action of this combination, in case of stomach disharmony, add *Zi Su Geng* (Caulis Perillae Frutescentis) and *Sha Ren* (Fructus Amomi). In case of stomach cold, add *Sheng Jiang* (uncooked Rhizoma Zingiberis) and *Sha Ren* (Fructus Amomi). In case of phlegm heat, add *Pi Pa Ye* (Folium Eriobotryae Japonicae). And, in case of stomach heat, add *Bai Mao Gen* (Rhizoma Imperatae Cylindricae) and *Pi Pa Ye* (Folium Eriobotryae Japonicae).

Bie Jia (Carapax Amydae Sinensis) & *Gui Ban* (Plastrum Testudinis)

Individual properties:	
Bie Jia	*Gui Ban*
Salty, slightly cold Turtle shell (dorsal carapax) Enriches yin and subdues yang Enriches yin and clears heat from the yin division Dispels stasis and scatters nodulations Usual dosage: 15-30g	Sweet, salty, neutral Land tortoise shell (primarily the ventral plastrum) Enriches yin and subdues yang Supplements the kidneys and strengthens bones Makes the heart & kidneys and *ren mai* & *du mai* communicate Usual dosage: 15-30g

Properties when combined:

When these two medicinals are combined together, they make yin and yang interact. In addition, together, they enrich yin and clear vacuity heat, subdue yang, extinguish wind, and stop tremors.[3]

Major indications of the combination:

1. Tidal fever, steaming bones, and night sweats due to vacuity heat caused by yin vacuity (1)
2. Weakness of the limbs, involuntary trembling of the hands and feet, and a red tongue with little or no fur due to a warm disease which has damaged the fluids and which causes internal wind of the vacuity type (2)
3. Headaches, vertigo, head distention, and tinnitus due to ascendant hyperactivity of liver yang (2)
4. Hypertension due to yin vacuity which causes yang to rise (3)
5. Abdominal conglomeration, such as hepatomegaly and splenomegaly (4)

Notes:

(1) For these indications, uncooked *Bie Jia* and

vinegar dip-calcined *Gui Ban* should be prescribed

(2) For these indications, this combination is present in *San Jia Fu Mai Tang* (Three Shells Restore the Pulse Decoction). For these indications, uncooked *Bie Jia* and uncooked *Gui Ban* should be prescribed.

(3) For these indications, uncooked *Bie Jia* and uncooked *Gui Ban* should be prescribed.

(4) For these indications, vinegar dip-calcined *Bie Jia* and uncooked *Gui Ban* should be prescribed.

Comments:

(a) *Bie Jia* and *Gui Ban* enrich yin, subdue yang, and clear vacuity heat. They treat the branch (vacuity heat, hyperactivity of yang) and root (yin vacuity) simultaneously. However, *Bie Jia* is superior for clearing vacuity heat and *Gui Ban* for subduing yang.

(b) *Bie Jia* is incompatible with peach and amaranth (eaten in China as a vegetable).

---

[3]   Wiseman gives check tetany for *zhi jing*. We prefer stop tremors, spasms, or convulsions.

Bing Lang (Semen Arecae Catechu) & *Mu Xiang* (Radix Auklandiae Lappae)

Individual properties:	
Bing Lang	**Mu Xiang**
Acrid, bitter, downbearing Breaks & downbears the qi Frees the flow of the stools Disperses food stagnation Usual dosage: 10-12g	Acrid, warm, fragrant, draining Moves the qi Stops pain Disperses food stagnation Usual dosage: 5-10g

Properties when combined:

When these two medicinals are combined together, they effectively move the qi, disperse food stagnation, and stop pain.

Major indications of the combination:

1. Lack of appetite, no desire for food, abdominal and epigastric distention and pain aggravated by pressure, difficult defecation or dry stools due to a food stagnating in the stomach and intestines (1) (2)
2. Dysentery or diarrhea with tenesmus and abdominal pain due to qi stagnation (2) (3)
3. Constipation or difficult defecation due to qi stagnation (4)

Notes:

(1) For these indications, stir-fried till scorched *Bing Lang* and uncooked *Mu Xiang* should be prescribed. Food accumulation transforms into heat and damages fluids in the intestines. This, in turn, causes dry stools and difficult defecation.

(2) For these indications, this combination is used in *Mu Xiang Bing Lang Wan* (Auklandia & Areca Pills).
(3) For these indications, stir-fried till scorched *Bing Lang* and roasted *Mu Xiang* should be prescribed.
(4) For these indications, stir-fried till scorched *Bing Lang* and uncooked *Mu Xiang* should be prescribed.

Comment:

(a) *Mu Xiang* moves the qi and disperses food stagnation. This is the reason why it is often added to formulas supplementing the qi, blood, or yin in order to facilitate the assimilation of rich substances which are heavy to digest and in order to prevent qi stagnation (*i.e.*, loss of appetite, abdominal or epigastric distention, rumbling noises in the stomach, loose stools, or diarrhea). Thus it can be added to this type of formula whenever a concomitant spleen vacuity is suspected.

Bing Lang (Semen Arecae Catechu) & Nan Gua Zi (Semen Cucurbitae Moschatae)

Individual properties:	
Bing Lang	**Nan Gua Zi**
Kills parasites Downbears the qi and frees the flow of the stools Expels the head (*i.e.*, hook) of tapeworms Usual dosage: 15-100g	Kills parasites Expels the body of tapeworms Usual dosage: 30-120g

Properties when combined:

When these two medicinals are combined together, they effectively expel the head and the body of tapeworms.

Major indications of the combination:

1. Intestinal parasites, particularly tapeworms (1)

Note:

(1) In clinical practice, a decoction of *Bing Lang*

and *Nan Gua Zi* is prescribed to kill a tapeworm. Two hours after drinking this decoction, a decoction of *Da Huang* (Radix Et Rhizoma Rhei), 10-20g, is taken to precipitate the dying worms via defecation.

Comment:

(a) *Bing Lang* has an anaesthetizing effect on intestinal parasites since it quiets worms. This is particularly interesting in cases of abdominal pain caused by parasitosis.

Bu Gu Zhi (Fructus Psoraleae Corylifoliae) & Hu Tao Ren (Semen Juglandis Regiae)

Individual properties:	
Bu Gu Zhi	**Hu Tao Ren**
Supplements the kidneys and invigorates yang Promotes the intake of qi (by the kidneys) Strengthens true yang Warms the cinnabar field Warms the spleen and stops diarrhea Usual dosage: 6-10g	Supplements the kidneys and invigorates yang Constrains the lung qi, warms the lungs, calms or levels asthma Warms and supplements the life gate Moistens the intestines and frees the flow of the stools Usual dosage: 6-10g

Properties when combined:

When these two medicinals are combined together, they supplement metal and water. Therefore, together, they effectively constrain the lung qi and promote the intake of qi by the kidneys, stop cough and calm asthma.

Major indications of the combination:

1. Cough, dyspnea, and asthma due to kidney yang vacuity (1)
2. Lumbago, impotence, seminal emission, constipation, frequent and abundant urination, and enuresis due to kidney qi vacuity (1)

Note:

(1) For these indications, salt-processed *Bu Gu Zhi* should be prescribed.

Comments:

(a) Breathing is managed by two viscera: the lungs and the kidneys. The lungs govern the qi. It is the lungs which breathe in the air and send it down to the kidneys. The kidneys intake the air (literally, grasp the qi) and retain it at that level. "To promote the intake of qi", therefore, is a therapeutic method that aims at supplementing the kidneys so that they may fulfill their function of taking in the qi during respiration. *Bu Gu Zhi*, *Chen Xiang* (Lignum Aquilariae Agallochae), and *Ci Shi* (Magnetitum) all have a reputation for promoting the intake of qi by means of the kidneys.

(b) Regardless of the cause of vacuity of the true yang, internal cold will develop if true yang becomes vacuous. Since cold has a contracting and congealing nature, such vacuity cold may result in blockage of the flow of yang qi in the lower burner. Since the free flow of yang qi plays a role in defecation, this may, in turn result in cold

pattern constipation. Also, the kidneys control the two yin (*i.e.*, the anus and urethra) as well as opening and closing, and thus they play an important role in the two excretions (*i.e.*, urination and defecation). If the life gate fire becomes weak, the kidneys may lose control of correct retention or excretion, causing diarrhea or constipation. In this type of imbalance, the therapeutical strategy aims at supplementing the kidneys and invigorating yang. The medical substances that supplement yang are warm or hot by nature and tend to dry organic liquids. These substances also induce intestinal dryness, which, as a consequence worsens the constipation. However, nature has quite naturally arranged everything well. We know three medicinal substances that invigorate the yang and warm the kidneys without drying it, moisten the intestines and free the flow of the stools. These substances are *Hu Tao Ren*, *Suo Yang* (Herba Cynomorii Songarici), and *Rou Cong Rong* (Herba Cistanchis Deserticolae).

(c) *Bu Gu Zhi* is incompatible with pork blood which may be an ingredient in blood pudding or blood sausage.

Bu Gu Zhi (Fructus Psoraleae Corylifoliae) & *Rou Dou Kou* (Semen Myristicae Fragrantis)

Individual properties:	
Bu Gu Zhi	*Rou Dou Kou*
Supplements the kidneys and invigorates yang Supplements the spleen and stops diarrhea Secures the essence and controls urination Especially supplements the kidneys Usual dosage: 6-10g	Warms the spleen and scatters cold Astringes the intestines and stops diarrhea Moves the qi and disperses distention Especially supplements the spleen Usual dosage: 6-10g

Properties when combined:

One is warming; the other is astringing. One supplements the kidneys; the other supplements the spleen.

When these two medicinals are combined together, they effectively supplement spleen and kidney yang, secure the intestines and stop daybreak or cock-crow diarrhea of dawn.

Major indications of the combination:

1. Chronic diarrhea due to spleen-kidney yang vacuity (1)
2. Daybreak diarrhea with abdominal pain and rumbling noises due to spleen-kidney yang vacuity (2)

Notes:

(1) For these indications, this combination is used in *Si Shen Wan* (Four Spirits Pills). For these indications, salt mix-fried *Bu Gu* Zhi and roasted *Rou Dou Kou* should be prescribed.

(2) For these indications, this combination is used in *Er Shen Wan* (Two Spirits Pills).

Comment:

(a) Cockcrow diarrhea is also called fifth watch diarrhea. It is a specific type of diarrhea. Although it may be caused by food accumulation, excessive consumption of alcohol, or liver fire, this type of diarrhea almost always has its origin in kidney yang vacuity. The ancients used to consider the kidneys and stomach as masters of the anal and urethral sphincters. It is the yang qi of these two organs that permits the control of these two openings. If either of these two become weak, frequent urination or diarrhea may appear. Moreover, once kidney yang is vacuous, it can no longer warm and sustain the spleen and stomach and particularly their transportation and transformation functions. This causes accumulation of dampness that can lead to loose stools or diarrhea. In addition, before dawn, yang qi is, by nature, weak, while yin cold is still plentiful. If the yang of the kidneys and stomach is already insufficient, they will be even weaker at this time. In that case, these two organs may not control the two sphincters adequately and this then causes diarrhea early in the morning. Therefore, this particular type of diarrhea most commonly results from the combination of three different but associated mechanisms.

Cang Er Zi (Fructus Xanthii) & *Xin Yi Hua* (Flos Magnoliae Liliflorae)

Individual properties:	
Cang Er Zi	*Xin Yi Hua*
Acrid, bitter, warm, draining, drying Diffuses the lung qi Dispels wind & wind dampness Opens the portals of the nose[4] Usual dosage: 6-10g	Acrid, warm, fragrant, draining Dispels wind and resolves the exterior Opens the portals of the nose Usual dosage: 3-6g

Properties when combined:

When these two medicinals are combined together, they effectively dispel wind , diffuse the lung qi, and open the portals of the nose.

Major indications of the combination:

1. Common cold with headache, nasal congestion, and runny nose due to wind cold (1)
2. Deep source nasal congestion with headache, nasal congestion, loss of smell, and turbid nasal phlegm (1)
3. Chronic or acute rhinitis, allergic rhinitis, hypertrophic rhinitis, sinusitis, parasinusitis, and frontal sinusitis (1)

---

4   Previously, Wiseman gave open the portals for *kai qiao*. Now he suggests open the orifices. However, orifice in English is typically only used in terms of body orifices, while *kai qiao* in Chinese is the common term for opening the windows. Therefore, we prefer to retain his earlier suggestion.

Note:

(1) *Cang Er Zi* and *Xin Yi Hua* are probably the two most efficient Chinese medicinal substances to treat all types of rhinitis or sinusitis. However, other medicinals are also renowned, for example *Huo Xiang* (Herba Agastachis Seu Pogostemi), *Xi Xin* (Herba Asari Cum Radice), *Bai Zhi* (Radix Angelica Dahuricae), and *E Bu Shi Cao* (Herba Centipedae), depending on the disease mechanisms at work. For these indications, this combination is present in *Cang Er Zi San* (Xanthium Powder). This formula can be used as the basis for treating rhinitis or sinusitis. However, it is very important to combine these two medicinals with the other appropriate medicinals based on pattern discrimination.

In case of wind cold, add *Xi Xin* (Herba Asari Cum Radice), *Huo Xiang* (Herba Agastachis Seu Pogostemi), and *Ma Huang* (Herba Ephedrae) and subtract *Bo He* (Herba Menthae Haplocalycis). In case of wind heat, add *Ju Hua* (Flos Chrysanthemi Morifolii), *Jin Yin Hua* (Flos Lonicerae Japonicae), and *Lian Qiao* (Fructus Forsythiae Suspensae). In case of gallbladder heat, add *Yu Xing Cao* (Herba Houttuyniae Cordatae Cum Radice), *Long Dan Cao* (Radix Gentiana Scabrae), and *Huang Qin* (Radix Scutellariae Baicalensis). In case of lung-spleen qi vacuity, add *Huang Qi* (Radix Astragali Membranacei), *Bai Zhu* (Rhizoma Atractylodis Macrocephalae), and *Dang Shen* (Radix Codonopsitis Pilosulae) and subtract *Bo He* (Herba Menthae Haplocalycis).

Comment:

(a) *Cang Er Zi* is incompatible with horse meat or pork.

Cang Zhu (Rhizoma Atractylodis) & *Huang Bai* (Cortex Phellodendri)

Individual properties:	
Cang Zhu	**Huang Bai**
Acrid, bitter, warm, drying, draining Upbearing (the clear) and downbearing (the turbid) Dispels wind and dries dampness (mainly in the middle burner and exterior) Fortifies the spleen and stops diarrhea Usual dosage: 6-10g	Bitter, cold, clearing, drying Sinking and downbearing Clears heat and dries dampness (mainly in the lower burner) Drains fire and resolves toxins Usual dosage: 6-10g

Properties when combined:

One is warm, while the other is cold.
One is drying; the other clears.
When these two medicinals are combined together, they complement and reinforce each other. Together, they effectively clear heat and dry dampness, disperse swelling and stop pain.

Major indications of the combination:

1. Wilting of the lower extremities with pain in the sinews and bones due to damp heat pouring downward to the lower part of the body (1)

2. Abnormal vaginal discharge, external vaginal itching, and cloudy, scanty urination due to damp heat (2)
3. Red, swollen, hot, painful joints due to wind, damp, heat impediment (3)

Notes:

(1) For these indications, this combination is present in *Er Miao San* (Two Marvels Powder). For these indications, uncooked *Cang Zhu* and salt mix-fried *Huang Bai* should be prescribed.

(2) For these indications, stir-fried till

scorched *Cang Zhu* and uncooked *Huang Bai* should be prescribed.

(3) For this indication, this combination is included in *Cang Zhu San* (Atractylodes Powder). For this indication, uncooked *Cang Zhu* and uncooked *Huang Bai* should be prescribed.

Comments:

(a) Despite the fact that *Cang Zhu* mainly treats cold dampness, it can treat damp heat if it is combined with bitter, cold medicinals. It is one of the most drying substances of the whole Chinese materia medica. It is strictly contraindicated in cases of dryness or yin vacuity (unless other moistening and enriching medicinals, such as *Mai Men Dong* [Tuber Ophiopogonis Japonici] and *Shi Hu* [Herba Dendrobii], are also prescribed).

(b) *Cang Zhu* is incompatible with black carp, peach, plum, and Chinese cabbage (*Brassica Chinensis* or *Brassica Pekinensis*).

Chai Hu (Radix Bupleuri) & *Huang Qin* (Radix Scutellariae Baicalensis)

Individual properties:	
Chai Hu	**Huang Qin**
Drains the liver	Clears heat and dries dampness
Resolves depression	Stops bleeding and quiets the fetus
Eliminates heat by harmonizing	Drains fire and resolves toxins
Upbears clear yang	Downbears turbid yin
Drains the evils located in the external part of the *shao yang* (1)	Drains the evils located in the internal part of the *shao yang* (1)
Usual dosage: 5-15g	Usual dosage: 5-10g

Properties when combined:

One dispels; the other one drains.
One upbears clear yang; the other downbears turbidity.
One dispels external evils; the other drains internal evils.
When these two medicinals are combined together, they harmonize the interior with the exterior, the *shao yang*, and liver and gallbladder. Together, they also clear the liver and resolve depression as well as clear and eliminate dampness and heat particularly in the liver and gallbladder.

Major indications of the combination:

1. Alternating fever and chills, a bitter taste in the mouth, dry throat, pain and fullness in the chest and lateral costal regions, nausea, and lack of appetite due to a *shao yang* pattern (2)(3)
2. Malaria due to a *shao yang* pattern (3)
3. Liver depression transforming into fire

Notes:

(1) These functions can also be explained as follows: *Chai Hu* dispels (floating, upbearing action) evils (heat) limited to the superficial part of the *shao yang*. *Huang Qin* drains (sinking, downbearing action) evil heat limited to the internal part of the *shao yang*.

(2) For these indications, this combination is included in *Xiao Chai Hu Tang* (Minor Bupleurum Decoction).

(3) For these indications, uncooked *Chai Hu* and uncooked *Huang Qin* should be prescribed.

Comments:

(a) This combination is remarkably effective for hepato-biliary disorders, such as acute or chronic hepatitis, biliary lithiasis, cholecystitis, and hepatomegaly due to liver-gallbladder heat.
(b) See comment (a) on the combination of *Ban Xia* and *Huang Qin* above.

Chai Hu (Radix Bupleuri) & Sheng Ma (Rhizoma Cimicifugae)

Individual properties:	
Chai Hu	*Sheng Ma*
Resolves the exterior and clears heat Courses the liver and resolves depression Upbears yang qi more moderately than *Sheng Ma* Upbears *shao yang* clear qi (liver-gallbladder) Frees the flow of qi on the left side of the body Usual dosage: 2-18g	Resolves the exterior and clears heat Out-thrusts eruptions Upbears yang qi more strongly than *Chai Hu* Upbears *yang ming* and spleen clear qi Frees the flow of qi on the right side of the body Usual dosage: 3-12g

Properties when combined:

One is for the left; the other for the right.
One enters the *shao yang*; the other the *yang ming*.
When these two medicinals are combined together, they complement and mutually reinforce each other. Together, they upbear liver, stomach, and spleen yang qi.

Major indications of the combination:

1. Uterine prolapse, rectal prolapse, gastric ptosis due to central qi fall (1)
2. Metrorrhagia and abnormal vaginal discharge due to central qi fall
3. Chronic diarrhea or chronic dysentery due to central qi fall (1)
4. Shortness of breath and dyspnea with feeling of oppression and downward falling of the lungs due to qi fall (2)

Notes:

(1) For these indications, this combination is used in *Bu Zhong Yi Qi Tang* (Supplement the Center & Boost the Qi Decoction).

(2) For these indications, this combination is used in *Sheng Xian Tang* (Upbear the Fallen Decoction).

Comments:

(a) *Sheng Ma* and *Chai Hu*, prescribed separately, do not upbear the qi efficiently. It is necessary to combine them with qi-supplementing medicinals, such as *Huang Qi* (Radix Astragali Membranacei), *Ren Shen* (Radix Panacis Ginseng), and *Bai Zhu* (Rhizoma Atractylodis Macrocephalae) for them to be really effective for this purpose. This is because one cannot raise what is lacking. Therefore, alone, *Chai Hu* and *Sheng Ma* do not upbear the qi. On the other hand, alone, *Huang Qi* does upbear the qi, but not for long. *Chai Hu* and *Sheng Ma* plus *Huang Qi* upbear the qi effectively and for long periods of time.

(b) For all these indications, one should prescribe stir-fried till scorched *Chai Hu* and honey mix-fried *Sheng Ma*.

(c) For all these indications, a small dosage of *Chai Hu* and *Sheng Ma* is sufficient, *i.e.*, 3-5g, unless one wants to simultaneously clear yin fire due to spleen vacuity from the head and face. In that case, one can use a larger dose of *Sheng Ma*, *i.e.*, 9-15g.

(d) It is important to note that hyperactivity due to liver yang in turn due to enduring liver depression/depressive heat is a pathological qi and is not the same as clear yang. In this case, liver yang counterflows upward, in part, because spleen vacuity is not able to upbear clear yang.

Chan Tui (Periostracum Cicadae) & Shi Chang Pu (Rhizoma Acori Graminei)

Individual properties:	
Chan Tui	**Shi Chang Pu**
Light, clearing, upbearing, draining Dispels wind heat Disinhibits the throat Diffuses the portals of the lungs and increases the voice Usual dosage: 3-6g	Aromatic, drying, opening Transforms phlegm dampness Arouses the spirit Opens the portals Usual dosage: 6-12g

Properties when combined:

When these two medicinals are combined together, they reinforce each other. They effectively arouse the spirit and open the portals.

Major indications of the combination:

1. Vertigo, tinnitus, and deafness due to obstruction of the clear portals (1)

Note:

(1) The clear portals are the organs of the senses: the two eyes, two ears, two nostrils, and the mouth, altogether seven portals. These are the windows of the spirit through which the spirit is made conscious of the external world and communicates with it.

Comments:

(a) *Shi Chang Pu* is very effective for opening and unblocking the portals or orifices. Some materia medica maintain that *Shi Chang Pu* opens the nine portals. The nine portals include the anus and urethra in addition to the seven enumerated above. It is particularly effective for sensory or psychological problems such as deafness, tinnitus, nasal obstruction, blurred vision, loss of consciousness, slow-wittedness, loss of memory, dementia, and psychoses.

(b) Besides the notes described above, *Chan Tui* has the big advantage of being one of the few medicinals within Chinese medicine which calms the liver and settles convulsions effectively but which is also not toxic even when used at high dosages (up to 30g/day), as opposed to *Quan Xie* (Buthus Martensis) and *Wu Gong* (Scolopendra Subspinipes). This is the reason why it is used currently in pediatrics and especially for vexation and agitation, insomnia, night crying, night fears, nightmares, and clonic convulsions or epilepsy.

(c) *Shi Chan Pu* is incompatible with meat and lamb's blood as well as Maltose (*Yi Tang*).

(d) For differences between *Shi Chang Pu*, *Jiu Jie Chang Pu*, fresh *Chang Pu*, and water *Chang Pu*, see comment (a) under the combination *Ci Shi* and *Shi Chang Pu* below.

Chen Pi (Pericarpium Citri Reticulatae) & He Zi (Fructus Terminaliae Chebulae)

Individual properties:	
Chen Pi	**He Zi**
Acrid, dissipating Rectifies and moves the qi Dries dampness and transforms phlegm Usual dosage: 6-10g	Sour, astringent, bitter, draining Secures and downbears the lung qi Disinhibits the throat and opens the voice Usual dosage: 3-10g

Properties when combined:

One dissipates, while the other astringes. When these two medicinals are combined together, they complement each other. Together, they effectively constrain the lung qi, rectify the qi, and increase the voice.

Major indications of the combination:

1. Hoarse voice, loss of voice, and chronic cough (vacuity type) with loss of voice and phlegm in the throat (1)

Note:

(1) For these indications, uncooked Chen Pi and uncooked He Zi should be prescribed. The use of He Zi is contraindicated in case of phlegm heat or repletion patterns.

Comment:

(a) He Zi is also called mirobolan, one of the main medicinal substances used in traditional Tibetan medicine.

Chen Pi (Pericarpium Citri Reticulatae) & Qing Pi (Pericarpium Citri Reticulatae Viride)

Individual properties:	
Chen Pi	**Qing Pi**
Acrid, dissipating, upbearing, floating, moderate (1) Rectifies and regulates the lung, spleen, and stomach qi Dries dampness and transforms phlegm Harmonizes the middle burner Rectifies the qi on the right side of the body Outer skin of the ripe fruit of the mandarin orange tree Usual dosage: 6-10g	Bitter, acrid, sour, draining, downbearing Sinking, drastic (1) Drains the liver and gallbladder qi Disperses lump glomus and food accumulations Moves the qi on the left side of the body Outer skin of the immature fruit of the mandarin orange tree Usual dosage: 3-10g

Properties when combined:

One is for the right, while the other is for the left.

One is upbearing; the other is downbearing.
One is floating, the other is sinking.
When these two medicinals are combined

together, they effectively soothe the liver and regulate the stomach, harmonize liver and spleen, harmonize liver and stomach, and rectify the qi and stop pain.

Major indications of the combination:

1. Epigastric and abdominal distention and pain, chest and lateral costal region distention and pain due to disharmony of the liver and spleen, liver and stomach, or a liver depression qi stagnation (2) (3)

Notes:

(1) Zhang Zi-he, the famous 12th century physician (1156-1228 CE) of the Southern Song dynasty, said:

> Chen Pi is upbearing and floating, goes to the lungs and spleen, influences the upper (part) and frees the flow. Qing Pi is downbearing and sinking, goes to the liver and gallbladder, influences the lower (part), and drains.

(2) For these indications, uncooked or stir-fried Chen Pi and vinegar mix-fried Qing Pi should be prescribed. For these indications, in case of disharmony of the liver and spleen, this pair is advantageously combined with Bai Shao (Radix Albus Paeoniae Lactiflorae), Chai Hu (Radix Bupleuri), and Bai Zhu (Rhizoma Atractylodis Macrocephalae).

(3) This pair is also sometimes prescribed to treat food accumulation in the stomach, diarrhea with abdominal distention due to liver-spleen disharmony, and premenstrual syndrome due to liver-spleen disharmony.

Comments:

(a) Chen Pi moves the qi, harmonizes the stomach, and dries dampness. This is why it is often added to formulas which supplement the qi, blood, or yin in order to ease the assimilation of rich medicinal substances which are heavy to digest and in order to avoid qi stagnation (i.e., loss of appetite, abdominal or epigastric distention, rumbling noises in the stomach, loose stools or diarrhea). It can be systematically added to this type of formula in all cases where a concomitant spleen vacuity is suspected.

(b) When the fruit which is the source of Qing Pi is small, the whole fruit is used. It is then called Xiao Qing Pi or Xin Qing Pi. When the fruit is big, only the outer skin is used. It is then called simply Qing Pi. In both cases, the fruit is immature.

(c) The moderate action of Chen Pi of moving the qi allows its use for longterm treatment. The drastic action of Qing Pi of breaking the qi contraindicates its long-term use.

(d) The drastic action of Qing Pi can be lessened by controlling the dosage as described in the saying:

> One qian, it rectifies the qi. Two qian, it moves the qi. Three qian, it breaks the qi.

One qian is equivalent to slightly more than 3g.

Chen Pi (Pericarpium Citri Reticulatae) & Sang Bai Pi (Cortex Radicis Mori Albi)

Individual properties:	
Chen Pi	**Sang Bai Pi**
Fortifies the spleen and harmonizes the stomach Dries dampness and transforms phlegm Rectifies the qi Tropism: spleen, lungs Usual dosage: 6-10g	Clears heat from the lungs Stops cough and calms asthma Disinhibits urination and disperses swelling Tropism: lungs Usual dosage: 6-10g

Properties when combined:

One transforms phlegm; the other drains the lungs
One prevents the production of phlegm; the other clears the lungs
When these two medicinals are combined together, they effectively clear the lungs and transform phlegm, rectify the qi, stop coughing, and calm asthma.

Major indications of the combination:

1. Cough and asthma due to lung heat with abundant yellow phlegm (1)

Note:

(1) To treat cough or asthma due to phlegm heat in the lungs, one must:
a. Clear heat from lungs. This is the function of *Sang Bai Pi*.
b. Transform phlegm. This is the function of *Chen Pi*.
c. Rectify the qi. This is the function of *Chen Pi*. See comment (a) for the pair *Ban Xia* and *Chen Pi* above.
d. Stop cough or asthma. This is the function of *Sang Bai Pi*.
e. Prevent the production of new phlegm. This is the function of *Chen Pi*.

If there is spleen weakness affecting the functions of movement and transformation, dampness accumulates and engenders phlegm. The lungs being the receptacle of the phlegm engendered by the spleen, phlegm disturbs the function of the lung qi (*i.e.*, diffusion and downbearing) and causes cough and asthma. *Chen Pi*, by fortifying the spleen, rectifying the qi and by drying dampness can prevent the production of new phlegm.

Chen Pi (Pericarpium Citri Reticulatae) & *Zhu Ru* (Caulis Bambusae In Taeniis)

Individual properties:	
Chen Pi	*Zhu Ru*
Acrid, warm Rectifies the qi and fortifies the spleen Harmonizes the stomach and downbears qi counterflow Dries dampness and transforms phlegm Usual dosage: 6-10g	Sweet, cold Clears heat Downbears qi counterflow and stops vomiting Transforms phlegm heat Usual dosage: 6-10g

Properties when combined:

One is warm, while the other is cold. When these two medicinals are combined together, they clear and warm simultaneously, eliminating mixed cold and heat in the stomach. Together, they effectively harmonize the stomach, downbear qi counterflow, and stop vomiting.

Major indications of the combination:

1. Nausea, vomiting, and epigastric and abdominal distention due to spleen-stomach vacuity mixed with cold and heat (1) (2)
2. Nausea and vomiting during pregnancy (1)

Notes:

(1) For these indications, this combination is used in *Ju Pi Zhu Ru Tang* (Orange Peel & Bamboo Decoction). *Ju Pi* and *Chen Pi* are the outer skin of the same fruit, *i.e.*, the mandarin orange. However, *Ju Pi* is the recent skin, while *Chen Pi* is the aged skin. (See note (1) of the pair *Ban Xia* and *Chen Pi*.) *Ju Pi* is very drying and acrid, more draining and irritating to the stomach. *Chen Pi* is moderate and more efficient. *Chen Pi* is preferred for use in clinical practice.

(2) When there is spleen-stomach vacuity with mixed heat and cold, in actuality, the spleen is vacuous and cold or at least benefits from the use of warm ingredients, and the stomach is hot and requires clearing with cold medicinals.

Chuan Bei Mu (Bulbus Fritillariae Cirrhosae) & *Xing Ren* (Semen Pruni Armeniacae)

Individual properties:	
Chuan Bei Mu	*Xing Ren*
Moistens the lungs Transforms phlegm Stops the cough Usual dosage: 6-10g	Diffuses the lung qi Downbears the lung qi Stops cough and calms asthma Moistens the intestines and frees the flow of the stools Usual dosage: 6-10g

Properties when combined:

One moistens, while the other downbears. When these two medicinals are combined together, they moisten while transforming phlegm, downbear the qi and stop cough.

Major indications of the combination:

1. Chronic cough and/or dry cough with little or no phlegm, difficulty expectorating, and dry throat due to lung vacuity

2. Relentless cough with expectoration of yellow phlegm due to external evils or an accumulation of phlegm heat in the lungs

Comments:

(a) There are two distinct types of *Bei Mu*: *Chuan Bei Mu* (Bulbus Fritillariae Cirrhosae) and *Zhe Bei Mu* (Bulbus Fritillariae Thunbergii). The first one is mainly grown in Sichuan province, the other, in Zhejiang province. *Chuan Bei Mu* is small (a little bigger than a pea, about 0.5-1cm in diameter) and topped by a protuberance which also gives it the name *Jian Bei Mu* (pointed *Bei Mu*). *Zhe Bei Mu* is big (like a cherry, about 2-2.5cm in diameter). This also gives it the name of *Da Bei Mu* (large *Bei Mu*). The two *Bei Mu* both clear the lungs, transform phlegm and stop cough. But *Chuan Bei Mu*, which is sweet and cool, tends to moisten the lungs and treat enduring cough of the yin vacuity or dry heat types. This manifests as a dry, weak cough, difficult to expectorate phlegm, possibly bloody phlegm, dry throat, etc. *Zhe Bei Mu*, which is bitter, acrid, and cold, tends to clear heat and treat acute cough of the replete or external types, *i.e.,* a loud cough with profuse, thick, yellow phlegm.

(b) Because the price of *Chuan Bei Mu* is comparatively high, one can also prescribe the powder: *Chuan Bei Fen* (or *Chuan Bei Mian*). Dosage: 2-3g washed down by the decoction.

(c) There are two types of *Xing Ren. Ku Xing Ren* (bitter *Xing Ren*), also called *Bei Xing Ren* (northern *Xing Ren*), is the most frequently prescribed clinically. Its taste is bitter, its nature is warm, and it is downbearing and draining. It is slightly toxic. It is advantageously used for asthma or cough of the replete type, whether internal or external, and influenza or colds accompanied by cough with abundant phlegm. *Tian Xing Ren* (sweet *Xing Ren*) is also called *Nan Xing Ren* (southern *Xing Ren*). Its taste is sweet, its nature is neutral, and it is moistening (to the lungs and intestines). It is not toxic. It is favorably used for asthma and cough of the vacuity type and constipation of the dry type.

(d) It should be noted that the slight toxicity of *Xing Ren* due to the presence of arsenic is located in the superficial skin and tip of the seed. The preparation of *Dan Xing Ren* or scalded Armeniaca, by removing the tip and skin, considerably reduces the risks of toxicity.

Chuan Bei Mu (Bulbus Fritillariae Cirrhosae) & *Zhi Mu* (Rhizoma Anemarrhenae Aspheloidis)

Individual properties:	
Chuan Bei Mu	**Zhi Mu**

Sweet, bitter, cool
Tropism: upper burner: lungs, heart
Moistens the lungs
Transforms phlegm
Stops cough
Usual dosage: 6-10g
	Bitter, cold
	Tropism: upper burner: lungs
	    middle burner: stomach
	    lower burner: kidneys
	Enriches yin and moistens dryness
	Clears heat and drains fire
	Usual dosage: 6-12g

Properties when combined:

When these two medicinals are combined together, they effectively clear and moisten the lungs, enrich yin and drain fire, transform phlegm and stop cough.

Main indications of the combination:

1. Enduring dry cough with little phlegm and difficult expectoration, sometimes fever, dry mouth, and a dry, red tongue due to water vacuity causing rising fire or due to lung yin vacuity (1)
2. Cough due to lung heat which causes lung dryness (1)

Note:

(1) For these indications, this combination is used in *Er Mu San* (Two Mu Powder). For these indications, stir-fried *Zhi Mu* should be prescribed.

Chuan Lian Zi (Fructus Meliae Toosendan) & *Yan Hu Suo* (Rhizoma Corydalis Yanhusuo)

Individual properties:	
Chuan Lian Zi	*Yan Hu Suo*
Bitter, cold, downbearing, draining Clears & eliminates dampness & heat and clears the liver Moves the qi and stops pain Works in the qi division Usual dosage: 6-10g	Acrid, warm, dissipating, and frees the flow Quickens the blood and dispels stasis Rectifies the qi and stops pain Works in the blood division Usual dosage: 6-15g

Properties when combined:

One is for the qi, while the other is for the blood. One drains heat from the qi; the other moves the blood and dispels stasis.
When these two medicinals are combined together, they effectively clear heat and eliminate dampness, course the liver and move the qi, quicken the blood and stop pain.

Major indications of the combination:

1. Pain in the chest, epigastrium, abdomen, and lateral costal regions due to liver depression qi stagnation sometimes associated with liver blood stasis (1) (2)
2. Liver depression qi stagnation transforming into liver heat or fire (1)
3. Dysmenorrhea and menstrual irregularities due to qi stagnation and/or blood stasis (1) (3)
4. Heart pain due to qi stagnation and blood stasis (1) (2)

5. Inguinal hernia or diseases of the scrotum or testicles due to qi stagnating in the liver channel (1) (3)
6. Hepatitis, cholecystitis, and angiocholitis due to damp heat in the liver and gallbladder (1) (3)

Notes:

(1) For these indications, this combination is used in *Jin Ling Zi San* (Melia Powder). This formula is a major analgesic which can be systematically added to other prescriptions when pain is a key manifestation of the disorder and especially if this pain is due to qi stagnation and blood stasis. Thus, this formula can serve as a basis for treatments of pain due to qi stagnation and blood stasis. Modifications of *Jin Ling Zi San*: If there is headache, add *Chuan Xiong* (Radix Ligustici Wallichii) and *Hong Hua* (Flos Carthami Tinctorii). If there is chest pain, add *Jie Geng* (Radix Platycodi Grandiflori), *Zhi Ke* (Fructus Citri Aurantii), and *Xie Bai* (Bulbus Allii). If

there is lateral costal pain, add *Chai Hu* (Radix Bupleuri) and *Yu Jin* (Tuber Curcumae). If there is stomach and epigastric pain, add *Mu Xiang* (Radix Auklandiae Lappae) and *Dan Shen* (Radix Salviae Miltiorrhizae). If there is lower abdominal pain, add *Mu Xiang* (Radix Auklandiae Lappae) and *Tao Ren* (Semen Pruni Persicae). If there is lower abdominal pain occurring on the sides of the abdomen in the area traversed by the liver channel, add *Wu Yao* (Radix Linderae Strychnifoliae) and *Xiao Hui Xiang* (Fructus Foeniculi Vulgaris).

(2) For these indications, stir-fried till scorched *Chuan Lian Zi* and wine mix-fried *Yan Hu Suo* should be prescribed.

(3) For these indications, stir-fried till scorched *Chuan Lian Zi* and vinegar mix-fried *Yan Hu Suo* should be prescribed.

Comments:

(a) *Yan Hu Suo* is a strong analgesic that can be prescribed for any pattern of pain. When this medicinal is used by itself or with small dosages of other medicinals, its dosage should be raised up to 50g in decoction or 10g in powder.

(b) Originally, Rhizoma Corydalis was named *Xuan Hu Suo*. However, in ancient China, it was forbidden to bear the same name as the emperor. Thus, during the Northern Song dynasty, under the ruling of Zhen Zong, *Xuan Hu Suo* was renamed *Yan Hu Suo*. During the Qing dynasty, under the rule of Kang Xi, *Xuan Hu Suo* was renamed *Yuan Hu Suo*. This is the reason why these three synonyms are frequently seen in the ancient as well as contemporary materia medica.

Chuan Xiong (Radix Ligustici Wallicii) & *Dang Gui* (Radix Angelicae Sinensis)

Individual properties:	
Chuan Xiong	***Dang Gui***
Acrid, warm, upbearing, dissipating, drying Moves the qi and quickens the blood Treats the qi within the blood Dispels stasis and stops pain In the upper body, it goes towards the head & eyes In the lower body, it goes towards the sea of blood (*i.e.*, the uterus) (1) Mainly quickens the blood Dispels wind and stops pain Usual dosage: 6-10g	Sweet, acrid, warm, moving, moistening Nourishes the blood and quickens the blood Treats the blood within the blood Harmonizes the blood Regulates menstruation and stops pain Dispels stasis and disperses swelling Mainly nourishes the blood Moistens the intestines and frees the flow of the stools Usual dosage: 6-10g

Properties when combined:

One quickens the blood; the other nourishes the blood.

When these two medicinals are combined together, they move the qi and quicken the blood without damaging the blood. Conversely, they nourish the blood without producing stasis. In addition, they dispel stasis and stop pain.

Major indications of the combination:

1. Menstrual irregularities, dysmenorrhea, and postpartum abdominal pain due to blood stasis that may be mixed with qi stagnation (2)
2. Rheumatic pain due to wind dampness and blood vacuity
3. Headaches due to blood vacuity and/or blood stasis (3)
4. Wounds, ulcers, or enduring cutaneous inflammations due to qi and blood vacuity with qi stagnation and blood stasis (4)

Notes:

(1) Depending upon its context, the sea of blood may designate any of four different things: 1) the *chong mai*; 2) the liver; 3) the uterus; or 4) the acupuncture point *Xue Hai* (Sp 10).

(2) For these indications, this combination is present in *Xiong Gui San* (Ligusticum & Dang Gui Powder).

(3) For these indications, this combination is included in *Jia Wei Si Wu Tang* (Added Flavors Four Materials Decoction).

(4) For these indications, this combination is used in *Tou Nong San* (Out-thrust Pus Powder).

Comments:

(a) For all these indications as a whole, one should prescribe wine-processed *Chuan Xiong* and wine-processed *Dang Gui*. Uncooked *Chuan Xiong* may also be used in case of headaches or dermatological problems.

(b) Three therapeutic strategies are used in order to supplement the blood: 1) Supplement the blood & supplement the qi: The spleen is the origin of the engenderment and transformation of the qi and blood. In order to increase the production of blood, spleen qi must be supplemented. This strategy is particularly used when blood vacuity is due to qi vacuity. (See the pair *Dang Gui* and *Huang Qi*.) 2) Supplement the blood & move the qi: The majority of medicinal substances which nourish the blood are rich, slimy, and difficult to digest. They sometimes cause qi stagnation and produce dampness with loss of appetite, stomach rumbling, epigastric and abdominal distention, loose stools, etc. In that case, it is advised to add medicinals which fortify the spleen, dry dampness, and rectify the qi, such as *Chen Pi* (Pericarpium Citri Reticulatae), *Sha Ren* (Fructus Amomi), and *Mu Xiang* (Radix Auklandiae Lappae). (See the pair *Sha Ren* and *Shu Di*.) 3) Supplement the blood & quicken the blood: Supplementing the blood tends to "inflate" it, "thicken" it, and, therefore, to engender blood stasis.[5] This is why, when we want to vigorously nourish the blood, medicinals which quicken the blood should be added to avoid the creation of blood stasis. This is one of the advantages of the combination of *Chuan Xiong* and *Dang Gui*.

(c) *Dang Gui* is probably the best Chinese medicinal for treating blood stasis due to blood vacuity or accompanied by blood vacuity.

(d) *Dang Gui*, or rather *quan* or whole *Dang Gui*, harmonizes the blood. Harmonizing the blood is a term which, in the Chinese materia medica, is almost specific to *Dang Gui*. This is because *Dang Gui* is one of the few medicinal substances which nourishes and moves the blood simultaneously. This characteristic allows *Dang Gui* to nourish the blood without causing blood stasis. Other medicinals, such as *Ji Xue Teng* (Caulis Milletiae Seu Spatholobi), *Dan Shen* (Radix Salviae Miltiorrhizae), and *Hong Hua* (Flos Carthami Tinctorii), may pretend to possess this same combination of functions. However,

---

[5] Because these words are based on my Chinese teachers' oral lectures, I am not sure of their characters and, therefore, their technical translation.

their supplementing action on the blood is weak, particularly *Hong Hua's* (which nourishes the blood if it is used in small quantity, but which then loses its efficacy for dispelling stasis).

(e) *Chuan Xiong* treats the qi within the blood. This expression means that *Chuan Xiong* simultaneously moves the qi and the blood, that it addresses mainly the qi which then moves blood, and that it avoids the risk of blood stasis when blood is being nourished.

Chuan Xiong (Radix Ligustici Wallichii) & *Shi Gao* (Gypsum Fibrosum)

Individual properties:	
Chuan Xiong	**Shi Gao**
Acrid, warm, fragrant, dissipating, upbearing Moves the qi and quickens the blood Dispels wind and stops pain In the upper part of the body, it is directed toward head and eyes. Usual dosage: 6-10g	Sweet, acrid, cold, heavy, draining Clears heat from the qi division Drains internal heat Eliminates heat from the muscle aspect and from the exterior Usual dosage: 30-60g

Properties when combined:

One is for the blood, while the other is for the qi.
One is warm; the other is cold.
One dissipates; the other drains.
When these two medicinals are combined together, they dispel wind, clear and drain heat, quicken the blood and move the qi, and stop pain.

Major indications of the combination:

1. Headaches due to wind heat or replete heat (particularly that which is located on the *shao yang* or *jue yin* channels) (1)

Note:

(1) For this indication, uncooked *Chuan Xiong* and uncooked *Shi Gao* should be prescribed. For wind heat headache, combine these with medicinals which dispel wind.

Comments:

(a) *Chuan Xiong* is mainly indicated for wind dampness and wind cold headaches. However, it can be prescribed for all kinds of headaches if combined with other medicinal substances specific for the pattern. For example: For wind damp headache, add *Qiang Huo* (Radix Et Rhizoma Notopterygii) and *Bai Zhi* (Radix Angelicae Dahuricae). For wind cold headache, add *Fang Feng* (Radix Ledebouriellae Divaricatae) and *Jing Jie* (Herba Schizonepetae Tenuifoliae). For wind heat headache, add *Ju Hua* (Flos Chrysanthemi Morifolii) and *Bo He* (Herba Menthae Haplocalycis). For blood stasis headache, add *Hong Hua* (Flos Carthami Tinctorii) and *Yan Hu Suo* (Rhizoma Corydalis Yanhusuo). For blood vacuity headache, add *Dang Gui* (Radix Angelicae Sinensis) and *Ji Xue Teng* (Caulis Milletiae Seu Spatholobi). For replete heat headache, add *Shi Gao* (Gypsum Fibrosum) and *Zhi Mu* (Rhizoma Anemarrhenae Aspheloidis). For qi stagnation headache, add *Chai Hu* (Radix Bupleuri) and *Bai Ji Li* (Fructus Tribuli Terrestris). For liver yang hyperactivity headache, add *Tian Ma* (Rhizoma Gastrodiae Elatae) and *Huai Niu Xi* (Radix Achyranthis Bidentatae).

(b) To obtain the highest degree of efficacy from *Shi Gao*, its powdered form should be used to make the decoction.

Ci Shi (Magnetitum) & *Shi Chang Pu* (Rhizoma Acori Graminei)

Individual properties:	
Ci Shi	*Shi Chang Pu*
Enriches the kidneys and calms the liver Subdues yang and quiets the spirit Sharpens the hearing Usual dosage: 15-30g	Arouses the spirit and quiets the spirit Diffuses impediment Opens the portal or orifices Usual dosage: 6-10g

Properties when combined:

One enriches, while the other opens.
When these two medicinals are combined together, they enrich the kidneys and calm the liver, diffuse impediment and open the portals, and sharpen the hearing.

Major indications of the combination:

1. Tinnitus and/or deafness due to yin vacuity or vacuity fire caused by yin vacuity (1)
2. Headaches, vertigo, heart palpitations, vexation and agitation, and insomnia due to yin vacuity causing yang hyperactivity (2)

Notes:

(1) For these indications, vinegar dip-calcined *Ci Shi* should be prescribed.

(2) For these indications, uncooked *Ci Shi* should be prescribed. It is important to know that, unlike its vinegar dip-calcined form, uncooked *Ci Shi* can cause abdominal pain. This is why the dosage should be more moderate (15g) and why it must be systematically combined with *Shen Qu* (Massa Medica Fermentata) which enables the "digestion of metals."

Comments:

(a) *Shi Chang Pu* is a generic name which, in fact, covers three distinct medicinal substances. Despite the fact that these three medicinals have a similar general action, each has its particularity. *Jiu Jie Chang Pu* (Anemone Altaica Fish) transforms phlegm, eliminates phlegm wind, and opens the orifices. *Xian Chang Pu* or *Xi Ye Chang Pu* (Acorus Gramineus Soland Var. Pulsillus) is prescribed fresh (*xian*) and clears heat, transforms phlegm heat, and is used for loss of consciousness due to febrile disease or accumulation of phlegm fire. *Shi Chang Pu* (Acorus Gramineus Soland) transforms phlegm, eliminates dampness, and stimulates hunger. Moreover, the majority of importers of Chinese medicinals, substitute *Bai Chang Pu* or *Shui Chang Pu* (Acorus Calamus L.) for *Shi Chang Pu*. This has a similar action to that of *Shi Chang Pu* but without its same power. To treat sensory or psychological disorders due to phlegm confounding the orifices of the heart, *Jiu Jie Chang Pu* is the most appropriate and effective of these various medicinals.

(b) *Shi Chang Pu* is incompatible with meat, lambs blood, and Maltose (*Yi Tang*).

Da Huang (Radix Et Rhizoma Rhei) & Fu Zi (Radix Lateralis Praeparatus Aconiti Carmichaeli)

Individual properties:	
Da Huang	**Fu Zi**
Bitter, cold, precipitating	Acrid, hot, warming
Precipitates the stools	Warms the interior and invigorates yang
Disperses accumulations	Drains cold and rescues yang
Operates within the blood division	Operates within the qi division
Usual dosage: 6-10g	Usual dosage: 6-10g

Properties when combined:

One is cold, while the other is hot.
One drains; the other supplements.
One clears; the other warms.
One precipitates accumulation; the other drains cold.
One operates within the blood division; the other within the qi division.
When these two medicinals are combined together, they complement each other. Together, they warm the interior, precipitate accumulation of cold, and evacuate the stools.

Major indications of the combination:

1. Constipation, abdominal pain, fear of cold, and cold limbs due to accumulation of internal replete cold (1)

Note:

(1) For these indications, this combination is present in *Da Huang Fu Zi Tang* (Rhubarb & Aconite Decoction). For these indications, uncooked *Da Huang* and bland *Fu Zi* should be prescribed.

Comments:

(a) The Western literature is rather confused concerning the differences between *Fu Zi, Tian Xiong, Wu Tou, Chuan Wu Tou,* and *Cao Wu Tou.* In fact, *Fu Zi, Tian Xiong,* and *Wu Tou* all come from the same plant. *Wu Tou* (Radix Aconiti Carmichaeli) is the mother root of the

plant. *Fu Zi* (Radix Lateralis Praeparatus Aconiti Carmichaeli) is the secondary lateral roots of *Wu Tou.* Literally, its Chinese name means "annexed child." When there is only one lateral root, the medicinal is then called *Tian Xiong,* which literally means "the celestial male" because this remedy is reputed to be very powerful. It has the same actions and indications as *Fu Zi.* However, *Wu Tou* is the generic term which groups together many varieties of Aconite (approximately 15), the two best known being *Cao Wu Tou* or *Cao Wu* (Radix Aconiti Carmichaeli or Radix Aconiti Kusnezofii). This comes from the northeastern provinces of Shanxi, Hebei, and Liaoning. It is wild Aconite and the most toxic. *Chuan Wu Tou* or *Chuan Wu* (Radix Aconiti Carmichaeli) is the cultivated Aconite mainly from Sichuan province. It is comparatively less toxic than *Cao Wu Tou.*

(b) *Fu Zi* is one of the most toxic substances in the Chinese materia medica. In order to control its toxicity and benefit from its therapeutic effects, it is important to respect the following recommendations: 1) Never orally administer unprepared Aconite. Always prescribe bland *Fu Zi,* blast-fried *Fu Zi,* or other known prepared varieties. This type of preparation considerably lessens the secondary effects of *Fu Zi.* 2) Submit *Fu Zi* to a long process of decoction (*i.e.,* not less than 1 hour). Heat destroys the toxicity of *Fu Zi.* 3) Boil *Fu Zi* with *Gan Cao* (Radix Glycyrrhizae), 6g, which has the reputation of reducing the toxicity of *Fu Zi.* 4) Before drinking a decoction containing *Fu Zi,* taste the decoction with the tip of the tongue. If this causes tingling or numbness of the tongue, the process of decoction should be extended until these effects disappear. 5) Before drinking a decoction containing *Fu Zi*, it is advisable to add honey which has the reputation of lessening the toxicity of *Fu Zi*. This precaution is optional if *Gan Cao* has already been used. 6) In the beginning of treatment, prescribe a small dose of *Fu Zi* which may then be progressively increased as necessary. With all these measures, the use of *Fu Zi*, even at relatively high dosages (10-15g), is totally free of toxic side effects. It is important to note that some Chinese practitioners prescribe *Fu Zi* at very high dosages (30-50g) without harmful side effects, and other practitioners use it even in heat patterns. However, those without much clinical experience in the use of *Fu Zi*, should nevertheless use this medicinal with caution and constraint, following the above six guidelines for its safe use.

(c) For the use of *Da Huang*, see the notes for paired *Da Huang* and *Mang Xiao* below.

(d) *Fu Zi* is incompatible with soy sauce and millet. *Da Huang* is incompatible with pork.

(e) This pair when combined with *Xi Xin* (Herba Asari Cum Radice), as in *Da Huang Fu Zi Tang*, has shown an interesting action in the treatment of cold damp *bi* or impediment with yang vacuity and blood stasis as well as for *bi* with an accumulation of heat in the stomach and intestines with persistent constipation. In the first case, it is necessary to prescribe wine mix-fried *Da Huang*. In the second case, one should prescribe uncooked *Da Huang*.

(f) It is noteworthy to mention that some practitioners believe that small doses (1-3g) of *Da Huang* can have supplementing effects and that this medicinal can be integrated into any formula that supplements the middle burner. However, this is probably an indirect effect. As it is said, the bowels function when they are freely flowing. The spleen cannot be fortified and healthy if the stomach and intestines are not free flowing. In addition, when the spleen becomes weak and, therefore, it loses its control over transportation and transformation, the stomach typically becomes hot due to accumulation and depression. Therefore, a small amount of *Da Huang* can address this accumulation and heat even if the main symptoms are those of spleen vacuity and there is no marked constipation.

Da Huang (Radix Et Rhizoma Rhei) & *Mang Xiao* (Mirabilitum)

Individual properties:	
Da Huang	*Mang Xiao*
Bitter, cold, discharging, precipitating Frees the flow of the stools and promotes defecation Quickens the blood and dispels stasis Drains fire and resolves toxins Disperses accumulations in the intestines (heat, damp heat, food) Usual dosage: 3-15g	Salty, cold, moistening, softening Moistens dryness, softens the hard, and frees the flow of the stools Clears heat and drains fire Disperses swelling, stops pain, disperses food accumulation (external use) Usual dosage: 6-15g

Properties when combined:

One frees the flow of the stools; the other softens the stools.
When these two medicinals are combined together, they complement each other and reinforce each other. Together, they effectively precipitate replete heat and internal accumulation and free the flow of the stools.

Major indications of the combination:

1. Constipation with hard, dry stools and abdominal pain which worsens with pressure due to heat accumulation in the *yang ming* bowels (1) (2)
2. Constipation with hard, dry stools, high fever, delirium and mental confusion, and dry, yellow tongue fur due to replete heat in the *yang ming* bowels (1) (2)
3. Chronic or severe constipation due to heat (2)

Notes:

(1) For these indications, this combination is present in *Da Cheng Qi Tang* (Major Order the Qi Decoction).

(2) For all these indications, uncooked *Da Huang* should be prescribed.

Comments:

(a) *Da Huang* is a major medicinal substance to precipitate heat, damp heat, and/or food accumulation in the intestines and to treat heat type constipation. However, it can be used for any type of constipation when combined with other medicinals specific for the pattern.

(b) *Da Huang*'s purgative action is drastic. Therefore, it should be controlled by the prescriber. One can adjust this medicinal's action by prescribing within the following parameters: In terms of dosage, up to 3g of *Da Huang* is lightly purgative and stimulates digestion. This is because bitterness in low doses stimulates the stomach. More than 3g, the higher the dose, the more purgative its effect is. There is a wide variability in the degree of sensitivity of patients to the purgative effects of *Da Huang*. Profuse diarrhea can occur with only 3g in certain patients, whereas constipation can resist a 12g dose in another patient. It is, therefore, advisable to be careful and to start treatment with a small dose, increasing it gradually as necessary until the ideal dosage is reached. *Da Huang* is a remarkable medicinal substance. Its use ought to be learned.

The method of preparation is also important for tailoring and adjusting the effects of *Da Huang*. Uncooked *Da Huang* allows a more powerful purgative effect. Wine mix-fried *Da Huang* is very slightly purgative. Carbonized *Da Huang* is not purgative. Likewise, the method administration of this medicinal plays its part. Powders or infusions have a very strong purgative effect. Decoction for 5 minutes also has a very strong purgative effect. Decoction for 30 minutes has a moderate purgative effect. And finally, depending on what *Da Huang* is combined with, one can increase or decrease its purgative effect. For instance, *Da Huang* plus *Man Xiao* has a strong purgative effect, while *Da Huang* plus *Gan Cao* (Radix Glycyrrhizae) has a moderate purgative effect.

(c) When *Da Huang* is prescribed, the patient may have foul-smelling stools, abdominal pain, and dark urine which all disappear when the treatment is stopped. These are all signs of heat and accumulation being discharged from the body.

Da Zao (Fructus Zizyphi Jujubae) & *Sheng Jiang* (Uncooked Rhizoma Zingiberis)

Individual properties:	
Da Zao	*Sheng Jiang*
Sweet, nourishing Supplements the middle burner & qi Nourishes the blood Harmonizes the action of other medicinal substances Usual dosage: 2-5 fruits	Acrid, moving Moves the qi Dispels wind cold Warms the middle burner Usual dosage: 5-10g

Properties when combined:

When these two medicinals are combined together, they move the defensive qi, nourish the constructive qi, and harmonize the constructive and defensive. They also fortify the spleen and harmonize the middle burner.

Major indications of the combination:

1. Perspiration, fear of wind, and fever due to disharmony between constructive and defensive qi (1)
2. Fatigue, lack of strength, abdominal pain, and lack of appetite due to disharmony between the constructive and defensive qi (2)

Notes:

(1) For these indications, this combination is present in *Gui Zhi Tang* (Cinnamon Twig Decoction).

(2) For these indications, this combination is present in *Xiao Jian Zhong Tang* (Minor Fortify the Center Decoction).

Comments:

(a) This pair is very frequently used in many formulas. These two medicinals help insure the proper assimilation of the active principles of other medicinal substances. *Da Zao* supplements the middle burner, while *Sheng Jiang* moves the qi and warms the middle burner. They also harmonize the action of other medicinals, *Da Zao* and *Gan Cao* being the two main harmonizing medicinals in Chinese medicine.

(b) Contrary to what is commonly understood, *Sheng Jiang* is not simply raw ginger. It is the rhizome of fresh and young ginger, while *Gan Jiang* (dry Rhizoma Zingiberis) is the older, more mature, and dry rhizome. In both cases, they are uncooked which is the technical meaning of the word *sheng* when applied to Chinese medicinals.

(c) *Sheng Jiang* is incompatible with horse meat.

Da Zao (Fructus Zizyphi Jujubae) & *Ting Li Zi* (Semen Lepidii)

Individual properties:	
Da Zao	**Ting Li Zi**
Sweet, nourishing, harmonizing Supplements the middle burner Supplements the qi Nourishes the blood Harmonizes & moderates the action of other medicinal substances Harmonizes & protects the stomach Usual dosage: 5 fruits	Acrid, draining, bitter, cold, sinking, downbearing Drains the lungs Expels phlegm and calms asthma Disinhibits urination Powerful and drastic therapeutic action which tends to damage yin and the stomach Usual dosage: 3-10g

Properties when combined:

When these two medicinals are combined together, they powerfully drain the lungs, disinhibit urination, and drastically evacuate phlegm without damaging yin and the stomach. Together, they downbear the qi and calm asthma.

Major indications of the combination:

1. Asthma, cough with stertor, wheezing, a swollen face, and oliguria due to accumulation of phlegm in the lungs (1)

Note:

(1) For these indications, this combination is present in *Ting Li Da Zao Xie Fei Tang* (Red Dates & Lepidium Drain the Lungs Decoction).

Comments:

(a) There are two types of *Ting Li Zi. Tian Ting Li* is sweet Lepidium coming from the southern provinces. Its taste is bland. Its draining and dispersing properties are moderate. It drains the lungs and expels phlegm without damaging the stomach. *Ku Ting Li*, bitter Lepidium, comes from the northern provinces. This is the most currently prescribed in clinical practice and the most effective. Its flavor is bitter. Its draining action is strong. It strongly drains the lungs and expels phlegm and can damage the stomach. Therefore, its combination with *Da Zao* is essential.

(b) In order to slow down the drastic action of (*Ku*) *Ting Li Zi*, one can use *Da Zao* as well as stir-fried till scorched *Ting Li Zi*.

(c) *Da Zao* is a medicinal that harmonizes. It is often used when *Gan Cao* is incompatible with some medicinal substances. This is the case with *Gan Sui* (Radix Euphorbiae Kansui), *Yuan Hua* (Flos Daphnis Genkwae), *Jing Da Ji* (Radix Euphorbiae Pekinensis), and *Hai Zao* (Herba Sargassii) or in case of edema, anuria, or hypertension.

Dan Dou Chi (Semen Praeparatum Sojae) & Zhi Zi (Fructus Gardeniae Jasminoidis)

Individual properties:	
Dan Dou Chi	**Zhi Zi**
Acrid, bitter, cold, dissipating Resolves the exterior and promotes perspiration Diffuses and out-thrusts external evils from the exterior Eliminates vexation Usual dosage: 6-10g	Bitter, cold, draining Drains heart, liver, lung, and stomach fire Clears heat toxins from the three burners Clears heat and eliminates vexation Usual dosage: 5-10g

Properties when combined:

One resolves; the other clears.
When these two medicinals are combined together, they unite to form the clearing and diffusing and out-thrusting method to eliminate evils from the exterior and interior. Together, they effectively promote perspiration, drain evils from the exterior, clear and out-thrust heat from the interior, and eliminate vexation due to replete heat.

Major indications of the combination:

1. Vexation and agitation, insomnia, and irritability during or after a warm disease (1)
2. External contraction of wind heat or a febrile disease

Note:

(1) For these indications, this combination is used in *Zhi Zi Chi Tang* (Gardenia & Prepared Soybean Decoction). For these indications, stir-fried clear (*Dan*) *Dou Chi* should be prescribed. See below.

Comments:

(a) *Zhi Zi* is known to be one of the bitterest medicinals in the whole Chinese materia medica along with *Long Dan Cao* (Radix Gentianae Scabrae), *Mu Tong* (Caulis Akebiae), and *Huang Lian* (Rhizoma Coptidis Chinensis). When this type of medicinal is prescribed, the bitterness of

the decoction has to be managed. See comment (a) of the pair *E Jiao* and *Huang Lian* below.

(b) The epicarpium of the Gardenia fruit (*Shan Zhi Ke*) moves the blood and clears external heat. The seeds of the Gardenia fruit (*Shan Zhi Ren*) clear internal heat. The seeds with the epicarpium are superior for draining lung fire. The seeds without the epicarpium are superior for draining heart fire.

(c) *Dan Dou Chi* is a fermented product of the black soybean (Semen Glycines Hispidae, *Hei Dou*) with other ingredients. According to the type of fermentation, one will get either clear or *Qing Dou Chi* (the *Dan Dou Chi* which clears) or warm or *Wen Dou Chi* (the *Dan Dou Chi* which warms). *Qing Dou Chi* is superior to clear heat and eliminate vexation. *Wen Dou Chi* is superior for resolving the exterior and promoting diaphoresis. Although *Wen Dou Chi* is warm in nature, it is used in and preferred for wind heat affections. The acrid and cool medicinal substances which drain wind heat are moderate diaphoretics. Therefore, the addition of *Wen Dou Chi* to a wind heat treating formula is in order to promote diaphoresis more strongly, its warm nature being controlled by the other cooling medicinals. This is why, for instance, this medicinal is included in *Yin Qiao San* (Lonicerae & Forsythia Powder).

Dan Nan Xing (Pulvis Arisaematis Cum Felle Bovis) & Xuan Fu Hua (Flos Inulae)

Individual properties:	
Dan Nan Xing	**Xuan Fu Hua**
Clears & transforms phlegm heat Extinguishes wind and settles convulsions Eliminates phlegm wind Usual dosage: 3-10g	Transforms phlegm and stops cough Diffuses the lung qi and calms asthma Downbears the qi and stops vomiting Usual dosage: 3-10g

Properties when combined:

One clears, while the other diffuses. When these two medicinals are combined together, they clear heat and transform phlegm, stop cough and calm asthma. Together, they also extinguish wind and wash away phlegm in the channels and network vessels.

Major indications of the combination:

1. Cough, asthma, and chest oppression due to phlegm damp obstruction, phlegm heat, or stubborn phlegm in the lungs (1)
2. Numbness in the limbs due to phlegm (wind) in the channels and network vessels (1)

Note:

(1) In case of absence of heat and in the presence of damp or cold patterns, processed *Tian Nan Xing* (Rhizoma Arisaematis) may be favorably prescribed instead of *Dan Nan Xing*.

Comments:

(a) Usually flowers have an upbearing, floating property. However, *Xuan Fu Hua,* on the contrary, downbears the qi and disinhibits urination (*i.e.,* has a downbearing property).

(b) *Xuan Fu Hua* (Flos Inulae) and *Xuan Fu Geng* (Caulis Inulae) have similar actions. However, *Xuan Fu Geng* is superior for downbearing the qi and disinhibiting urination, while *Xuan Fu Hua* is superior for dispersing phlegm, downbearing the qi, and calming asthma.

Dan Shen (Radix Salviae Miltiorrhizae) & Mu Dan Pi (Cortex Radicis Moutan)

Individual properties:	
Dan Shen	**Mu Dan Pi**
Quickens the blood and dispels stasis Cools the blood and clears heat Eliminates stasis and engenders new (tissue) Disperses swelling and stops pain Usual dosage: 10-15g	Quickens the blood and dispels stasis Clears heat, cools the blood, and clears the liver Eliminates vacuity heat lodged in the yin division Stops bleeding Usual dosage: 6-10g

Properties when combined:

Dan Shen quickens the blood more strongly, while *Mu Dan Pi* cools the blood more strongly. When these two medicinals are combined together, they complement and reinforce each other. Together, they effectively quicken the blood and dispel stasis, cool the blood and eliminate vacuity heat.

Major indications of the combination:

1. Hematemesis, epistaxis, metrorrhagia, purpura but also rubella, and pruritus due to heat in the blood division
2. Menstrual irregularities, dysmenorrhea, amenorrhea, dark purple menstrual blood with clots, and postpartum abdominal pain due to heat in the blood which causes blood stasis
3. Continuous, low-grade fever due to yin vacuity which causes vacuity heat (1)
4. Hot, red, swollen, painful joints due to heat *bi* or impediment

Note:

(1) For this indication, *Mu Dan Pi* is used if there are no night sweats. Otherwise, *Di Gu Pi* (Cortex Radicis Lycii Chinensis) should be used.

Comments:

(a) The ancients said: "A drink made of only *Dan Shen* is similar in effect to *Si Wu Tang* (Four Materials Decoction)." *Si Wu Tang* nourishes the blood and quickens the blood harmoniously. *Dan Shen* also quickens the blood and nourishes the blood. Nevertheless, *Si Wu Tang* and *Dan Shen* are distinct in the following aspects: 1) *Dan Shen* only moderately nourishes the blood and mainly quickens the blood. To reinforce its supplementing action, one must prepare *Dan Shen* with pig or tortoise blood. *Si Wu Tang* moderately moves the blood and mainly nourishes the blood. 2) *Dan Shen* has a cool nature and is, therefore, better adapted for heat patterns. *Si Wu Tang* is warm in nature and is, therefore, better for cold patterns. Therefore, in my opinion, the above saying is only meant to remind practitioners that *Dan Shen* not only quickens but also nourishes the blood if only moderately. It is not meant to be taken at full face value.

(b) *Dan Shen* is incompatible with vinegar or any other very sour or acrid food. *Mu Dan Pi* is incompatible with garlic and coriander.

Dan Shen (Radix Salviae Miltiorrhizae) & *San Qi* (Radix Pseudoginseng)

Individual properties:	
Dan Shen	*San Qi*
Quickens the blood and dispels stasis	Quickens the blood and dispels stasis
Eliminates stasis and genders new (tissue)	Stops bleeding
Disperses swelling and stops pain	Disperses swelling
Nourishes the heart and quiets the spirit	Stops pain
Usual dosage: 10-15g	Usual dosage: 3-10g (1)

Properties when combined:

When these two medicinals are combined together, they complement and reinforce each other. Together, they effectively quicken the blood and dispel stasis, nourish the heart and open the network vessels, stop pain and settle palpitations.

Major indications of the combination:

1. Chest *bi* or impediment, *i.e.*, cardiac problems with pain and severe palpitations (2)

Notes:

(1) There are two methods of preparing *San Qi*,

uncooked and steamed. Uncooked *San Qi* quickens the blood, dispels stasis, and stops bleeding. Steamed *San Qi* nourishes the blood and is not effective for either quickening the blood or stopping bleeding. If *San Qi* is cooked by adding it together with other decocting medicinals, its ability to quicken the blood and stop bleeding is lost. Therefore, for these indications, *San Qi* is more efficient when administered in its powdered form. Its dosage is then 1-3g.

(2) For these indications, wine mix-fried *Dan Shen* should be prescribed. This combination treats heart pain no matter what its cause. This action may be reinforced advantageously by combining *Dan Shen* with *Shi Chang Pu* (Rhizoma Acori Graminei), *Xie Bai* (Bulbus Allii), *Gua Lou Pi* (Pericarpium Trichosanthis Kirlowii), *Gui Zhi* (Ramulus Cinnamomi Cassiae), and *Tan Xiang* (Lignum Santali Albi).

Comment:

(a) Modern research has clearly demonstrated that *San Qi* has a definite effect on coronary heart disease, angina pectoris, and hypercholesterolemia and that *Dan Shen* also has a very interesting action on coronary heart disease, circulatory system diseases, and hypercholesterolemia.

Dan Shen (Radix Salviae Miltiorrhizae) & *Tan Xiang* (Lignum Santali Albi)

Individual properties:	
Dan Shen	*Tan Xiang*
Tropism: the blood division Dispels stasis Quickens the blood and stops pain Usual dosage: 10-15g	Tropism: the qi division Disperses qi stagnation Scatters cold and stops pain Usual dosage: 3-6g

Properties when combined:

One is for the blood, while the other is for the qi. When these two medicinals are combined together, they effectively regulate and rectify the qi and blood, move the qi and quicken the blood, free the flow of the network vessels and stop pain.

Major indications of the combination:

1. Chest *bi* or impediment, heart diseases with severe cardiac pain due to qi and blood stasis and stagnation (1) (2)
2. Stomach pain due to qi and blood stasis and stagnation (1)

Notes:

(1) For these indications, wine mix-fried *Dan Shen* should be prescribed.

(2) If heart blood stasis is severe, it is advantageous to add *San Qi* (Radix Pseudoginseng), *Hong Hua* (Flos Carthami Tinctorii), and *Yan Hu Suo* (Rhizoma Corydalis Yanhusuo). If qi stagnation is severe, it is advantageous to add *Chen Xiang* (Lignum Aquilariae Agallochae) and *Qing Mu Xiang* (Radix Aristolochiae). If, furthermore, there is phlegm damp obstruction in the chest, it is advantageous to add *Gua Lou Pi* (Pericarpium Trichosanthis Kirlowii), *Jie Geng* (Radix Platycodi Grandiflori), and *Zhi Ke* (Fructus Citri Aurantii). If, in addition, there is chest yang vacuity, it is advantageous to add *Xie Bai* (Bulbus Allii), *Gui Zhi* (Ramulus Cinnamomi Cassiae), and *Fu Zi* (Radix Lateralis Praeparatus Aconiti Carmichaeli). If, in addition, there is qi vacuity, it is advantageous to add *Huang Qi* (Radix Astragali Membranacei), *Zhi Gan Cao* (Radix Glycyrrhizae), and *Ren Shen* (Radix Panacis Ginseng).

Dang Gui (Radix Angelicae Sinensis) & Huang Qi (Radix Astragali Membranacei)

Individual properties:	
Dang Gui	**Huang Qi**
Nourishes the blood Quickens the blood Dispels blood stasis hindering the engenderment of new blood Usual dosage: 6-9g	Fortifies the spleen & middle burner Supplements the qi to engender and transform the blood and to control the blood Engenders muscles (*i.e.*, flesh) Usual dosage: 15-30g

Properties when combined:

One is for the blood; the other is for the qi. When these two medicinals are combined together, they supplement the qi to strongly engender and transform the blood. Therefore, they effectively supplement the qi and blood.

Major indications of the combination:

1. Delayed menstruation, *i.e.*, a long menstrual cycle, postpartum weakness, agalactia due to qi and blood vacuity (1)
2. Low-grade fever caused by blood vacuity (2)
3. Sores and welling abscesses which do not heal due to qi and blood vacuity (3)
4. Numbness of the limbs due to blood vacuity not nourishing the sinews
5. Various hemorrhages due to qi not containing the blood within the vessels (2)

Notes:

(1) For these indications, this combination is used in *Shi Quan Da Bu Tang* (Ten [Ingredients] Wholly & Greatly Supplementing Decoction).

(2) For these indications, this combination is used in *Dang Gui Bu Xue Tang* (Dang Gui Supplement the Blood Decoction).

(3) For this indication, this combination is used in *Tou Nong San* (Out-thrust Pus Powder).

Comments:

(a) For all these indications, one should prescribe wine mix-fried *Dang Gui* and honey mix-fried *Huang Qi*. Also, it is advised to use whole or *Quan Dang Gui* or the body of *Dang Gui* or *Dang Gui Shen*. (See the pair *Dang Gui* and *Shu Di* below.)

(b) When spleen's function of transformation is insufficient, this causes weak production of blood and, therefore, blood vacuity. This combination aims at strongly supplementing the qi to engender the blood. Thus it treats blood vacuity due to qi vacuity.

(c) Even if this pair treats blood vacuity, one should use a relatively light dosage of *Dang Gui*. Why? Because here blood vacuity is due to qi vacuity and weakness of the middle burner. Medicinals that nourish the blood, such as *Dang Gui*, tend to be rich, slimy, and difficult to assimilate in cases of spleen weakness. Therefore, a small dosage of *Dang Gui* is used to avoid damaging the spleen and causing further weakness, qi stagnation, and dampness engenderment which would lead to even worse production of blood. Furthermore, since the origin of blood vacuity is qi vacuity, the therapeutic strategy has to be first of all to supplement the qi and then the blood.

(d) The pairing of *Dang Gui* and *Huang Qi* in *Dang Gui Bu Xue Tang* is a typical example of the method of combining sweet and warm medicinals to treat fever. Blood, which is yin by nature, participates in the balancing of yin and yang. Hence, if there is blood vacuity, the harmony between yin and yang is broken. Yang is no longer anchored and tends to spread towards the exterior, causing vacuity heat with low fever, a red complexion, skin which is warm to the touch, and a big, vacuous, floating pulse. Wu Kun (1551-1620?), a famous physician of the Ming dynasty, said:

> When the blood is full, the body is cool. When the blood is vacuous, the body is warm.

Huang Qi strongly supplements the qi (yang) to engender the blood (yin), secures the exterior and returns floating yang qi back to its source. Thus, *Dang Gui* is combined with *Huang Qi* to engender and transform the blood. As said in the *Nei Jing (Inner Classic)*, "When yang engenders, yin grows" and, "When yin blood gradually is engendered, yang has someplace to which to attach." Thus there is a harmony between yin and yang.

Dang Gui (Radix Angelicae Sinensis) & *Shu Di* (Cooked Radix Rehmanniae)

Individual properties:	
Dang Gui	*Shu Di*
Nourishes the blood and balances the blood Quickens the blood and dispels stasis Mobile by nature Downbears the qi, stops cough, and calms asthma (1) Moistens the intestines and frees the flow of the stools Usual dosage: 6-10g	Nourishes the blood, yin, and essence Enriches the kidneys and nourishes the liver Fixed by nature Promotes the qi intake function of the kidneys and calms asthma Usual dosage: 6-15g

Properties when combined:

When these two medicinals are combined together, they nourish the blood and enrich yin, supplement the liver and kidneys. Together, they downbear the lung qi and promote the qi intake by the kidneys, stop cough and calm asthma.

Major indications of the combination:

1. Chronic cough and/or asthma due to yin vacuity of the kidneys associated with blood vacuity (2)
2. Blood vacuity (3)
3. Constipation due to blood vacuity (4)

Notes:

(1) This function, even if not very well known, is very real. It is quoted in ancient materia medica, such as the *Shen Nong Ben Cao Jing (The Divine*

Husbandman's Materia Medica Classic) and the *Ben Cao Hui Bian (Collected Materia Medica)*, and it is expressed in many formulas, among which the most famous is *Su Zi Jiang Qi Tang* (Perilla Seed Downbear the Qi Decoction). For this function, whole or *Quan Dang Gui* should be used. (See below.)

(2) If there is blood vacuity, qi lacks its root. This can create an imbalance in the upbearing and downbearing function of the qi with lung qi vacuity. If the kidneys are weak, they cannot insure their function of qi intake. This then results in qi counterflow and asthma. For these indications, this combination can be found in *Jin Shui Liu Jun Jian* (Metal & Water Six Gentlemen Decoction).

(3) This combination, which is included in *Si Wu Tang* (Four Materials Decoction), allows for the effective nourishment of the blood without

engendering blood stasis. This is due to the action of *Dang Gui* which quickens the blood.

(4) *Dang Gui* and *Shu Di* are probably the two most effective medicinal substances for treating constipation due to blood vacuity. One should keep in mind that *Dang Gui You*, the oil extracted from *Dang Gui* is particularly indicated for nourishing the blood and moistening dryness, moistening the intestines and promote defecation.

Comments:

(a) The action of *Dang Gui* is different according to the part used. *Dang Gui Tou*, the head of *Dang Gui*, is the superior extremity of the root. It quickens the blood and stops bleeding. This part is often prepared by stir-frying till carbonized to reinforce its hemostatic action. *Dang Gui Shen*, the body of *Dang Gui*, the main part of the root, nourishes the blood. *Dang Gui Wei*, the tails of *Dang Gui* or the secondary roots of the inferior extremity, quicken the blood and breaks blood stasis. This part is often wine-processed to reinforce its action of quickening the blood. *Dang Gui Xu*, the beard of *Dang Gui*, are the rootlets of the main and secondary roots. They quicken the blood and free the flow of the network vessels. This part is often prepared by wine-processing to reinforce its action of quickening the blood and freeing the flow of the network vessels. *Quan Dang Gui* corresponds to the entire root which includes the four parts previously mentioned. It quickens the blood and nourishes the blood. Therefore, it harmonizes the blood. (See comment (d) of the pair *Chuan Xiong* and *Dang Gui* above.) Li Dong Yuan (1180-1251), the famous author of the *Pi Wei Lun (The Treatise on the Spleen & Stomach)*, said of *Dang Gui*:

> The head stops bleeding and is directed upwards. The body nourishes the blood and is fixed to the center. The tails break the blood and flow downward. The whole root quickens the blood and treats everything.

(b) *Shu Di* is incompatible with animal blood whatever the animal, onions, chives, turnips, radishes, and garlic.

Dang Shen (Radix Codonopsitis Pilosulae) & *Huang Qi* (Radix Astragali Membranacei)

Individual properties:	
Dang Shen	*Huang Qi*
Supplements the spleen & stomach Supplements the qi and promotes the engenderment of blood and fluids Sweet, neutral, fixed, tends to supplement the middle burner & yin Usual dosage: 10-15g	Supplements the qi and upbears yang Secures the exterior and stops perspiration Promotes tissue regeneration Sweet, warm, mobile, tends to supplement the exterior & yang Usual dosage: 10-30g

Properties when combined:

One is for the interior; the other is for the exterior.
One is for the middle burner qi; the other is for the defensive qi.
One is for yin; the other for yang.
When these two medicinals are combined together, they powerfully supplement the qi. Together, they effectively supplement the qi of the middle burner and the exterior defensive.

Major indications of the combination:

1. Chronic illness leading to qi vacuity (1)
2. Rectal and uterine prolapse and gastric ptosis

due to central qi fall (1) (2)

3. Lack of appetite, loose stools, fatigue, lack of strength, and spontaneous perspiration due to qi vacuity (1)

4. Low-grade fever due to qi vacuity (2)

Notes:

(1) When one wants to supplement the middle burner, one should prescribe honey mix-fried *Dang Shen* and honey mix-fried *Huang Qi*. In case of loose stools or diarrhea, one should prescribe rice stir-fried *Dang Shen*. In case of spontaneous perspiration, one should prescribe uncooked *Huang Qi*.

(2) For these indications, this combination is included in *Bu Zhong Yi Qi Tang* (Supplement the Center & Boost the Qi Decoction).

Comments:

(a) *Dang Shen* does not directly nourish the blood and fluids. *Dang Shen* supplements the spleen which is the latter heaven or postnatal root, the origin of qi, blood, fluids and humors, and acquired essence.

(b) *Huang Qi* effectively upbears yang qi if it is combined with *Chai Hu* (Radix Bupleuri) and/ or *Sheng Ma* (Rhizoma Cimicifugae). See comment (a) of the pair *Chai Hu* and *Sheng Ma* above.

(c) *Huang Qi Pi* (Cortex Radicis Astragali Membranacei), the bark of the Astragalus root, goes to the exterior and is more powerful than *Huang Qi* for securing the exterior and stopping perspiration, disinhibiting urination and treating edema.

(d) The disease mechanism of fever due to yin vacuity or blood vacuity is easy to understand. (See comment (d) of the pair *Dang Gui* and *Huang Qi* above.) The disease mechanism associated with qi vacuity is less obvious. It can be explained in different manners, but all of these come down to an imbalance between yin and yang. For example, 1) in case of severe qi vacuity in the middle burner (yang), blood (yin) is not adequately produced and causes simultaneously qi and blood vacuity. This blood vacuity induces a yin-yang imbalance causing fever. 2) In case of severe qi vacuity, yang detaches itself from yin (yang desertion) causing floating yang and, therefore, fever. 3) Qi vacuity can lead to yang vacuity. Moreover, "diminished yang damages yin." This means that a weakening of yang can cause yin vacuity because of the intimate relation between yin and yang. Yin vacuity causes vacuity heat and, therefore, fever. 4) The spleen is the origin of the production of blood, fluids and humors, and the postnatal essence or the "acquired yin." Thus spleen qi vacuity over a long period can lead to kidney yin vacuity. In that case, kidney water can no longer control heart fire and the yin-yang balance is disturbed, causing fever. 5) In case of middle burner (yang) qi vacuity, the imperial fire (qi-yang) of the heart is not sufficient to descend and warm, activating kidney water. Kidney water then stagnates below and can no longer control heart fire above, causing fever.

Other disease mechanisms can also explain qi vacuity fever. This fever is classified among the fevers due to internal damage. In all cases, the origin of the trouble is a spleen qi vacuity. The spleen likes sweetness and fears bitter, likes warmth and fears cold, likes supplementation and fears dispersion, likes movement and fears stagnation, likes upbearing and fears downbearing, likes dryness and fears dampness. Therefore, the therapeutic strategy is to fortify the spleen qi by namely supplementing, upbearing, drying, moving, sweet, and warm medicinal substances in order to eliminate fever.

Bu Zhong Yi Qi Tang, in which the pair *Dang Shen* and *Huang Qi* is present, corresponds perfectly to this strategy. In terms of the sweet taste, it contains *Dang Shen* (Radix Codonopsitis Pilosulae), *Huang Qi* (Radix Astragali Membranacei), *Zhi Gan Cao* (mix-fried Radix Glycyrrhizae), *Bai Zhu* (Rhizoma Atractylodis Macrocephalae), and *Dang Gui* (Radix Angelicae Sinensis). In terms of warm natured medicinals, it contains *Dang Shen, Huang Qi, Zhi Gan Cao, Bai Zhu, Dang Gui,* and *Chen* Pi (Pericarpium Citri Reticulatae). As for qi-supplementing medicinals, it includes *Dang Shen, Huang Qi, Zhi Gan Cao,* and *Bai Zhu*. As for movement, *Chen*

Pi moves the qi, while *Dang Gui* moves the blood. As for upbearing, *Huang Qi, Sheng Ma* (Rhizoma Cimicifugae), and *Chai Hu* (Radix Bupleuri) all upbear yang qi. And in terms of drying, *Bai Zhu* and *Chen Pi* both are drying. Therefore, *Bu Zhong Yi Qi Tang* is the prototypical formula for "eliminating heat using sweet taste and warm nature."

Di Gu Pi (Cortex Radicis Lycii Chinensis) & *Sang Bai Pi* (Cortex Radicis Mori Albi)

Individual properties:	
Di Gu Pi	*Sang Bai Pi*
Tropism: kidneys, lungs & yin division Drains fire from the lungs Clears heat and cools the blood Eliminates vacuity heat Eliminates evils from the yin division Usual dosage: 10-15g	Tropism: lungs & qi division Clears the heat from the lungs without damaging the qi Calms asthma Disinhibits urination and disperses swelling without damaging yin Eliminates evils from the qi division Usual dosage: 6-10g

Properties when combined:

One is for the yin; the other for the qi. When these two medicinals are combined together, they clear the yin and qi divisions. Together, they effectively clear heat from the lungs, drain fire from the lungs, eliminate vacuity fire damaging the lungs, stop cough and calm asthma.

Major indications of the combination:

1. Cough and asthma with expectoration of yellow, sticky, and thick phlegm, fever, and thirst due to lung heat (1)
2. Cough accompanied by evening fever or low but persistent fever with skin which is warm to the touch due to vacuity heat damaging the lungs (1)

Note:

(1) For these indications, this combination is found in *Xie Bai San* (Drain the White Powder). For these indications, honey mix-fried *Sang Bai Pi* should be prescribed. In case of replete heat, it is advantageous to add *Huang Qin* (Radix Scutellariae Baicalensis), *Pi Pa Ye* (Folium Eriobotryae Japonicae) and *Zhe Bei Mu* (Bulbus Fritillariae Thunbergii). In case of vacuity heat, it is advantageous to add, *Zhi Mu* (Rhizoma Anemarrhenae Aspheloidis) and *Mai Men Dong* (Tuber Ophiopogonis Japonici).

Comment:

(a) What is interesting about this combination is the fact that it can treat both replete heat and vacuity heat of the lungs. It is important to note that the lungs are the delicate viscus and are easily damaged by heat. Replete heat easily damages lung yin, causing replete and vacuity heat simultaneously. The pair *Di Gu Pi* and *Sang Bai Pi* treats this situation very well.

Ding Xiang (Flos Caryophylli) & *Shi Di* (Calx Khaki)

Individual properties:	
Ding Xiang	*Shi Di*
Acrid, warm, dissipating Warms the center and stops hiccup and vomiting Scatters cold and stops pain Usual dosage: 3-6g	Bitter, neutral, astringent Downbears the qi Stops hiccup Usual dosage: 6-10g

Properties when combined:

One disperses, while the other moves downward. When these two medicinals are combined together, they complement each other. Together, they effectively warm the middle burner and scatter cold, downbear qi counterflow and stop hiccup.

Major indications of the combination:

1. Hiccup due to cold in the stomach (1)
2. Nausea and vomiting due to vacuity cold in the spleen and stomach (1)

Note:

(1) For these indications, this combination is present in *Shi Di Tang* (Persimmon Calx Decoction). For hiccup, it is useful to add *Chen Xiang* (Lignum Aquilariae Agallochae).

Comments:

(a) *Ding Xiang You*, the aromatic oil extracted from cloves, warms the stomach and scatters cold. Applied externally, it mainly treats epigastric pain, rheumatic pain, and toothache due to cold.

(b) Cloves are the flower bud of the clove tree. Some flowers are male; others are female. The male *Ding Xiang*, *Gong Ding Xiang* (literally, *Ding Xiang* father) is reputed to be more powerful than the female *Ding Xiang*, *Mu Ding Xiang* (literally, *Ding Xiang* mother).

Du Huo (Radix Angelicae Pubescentis) & Qiang Huo (Radix Et Rhizoma Notopterygii)

Individual properties:	
Du Huo	**Qiang Huo**
Tropism: the lower part of the body, lumbar area, knees, legs, feet & *shao yin* Moderate in action Dispels wind and resolves the exterior Eliminates wind dampness and treats *bi* Treats hidden wind or wind which is more internal and fixed. Usual dosage: 6-10g	Tropism: the upper part of the body, occiput, nape of the neck, shoulders, upper limbs & *tai yang* Powerful in action Drains wind, cold, and dampness and resolves the exterior Eliminates wind dampness and treats *bi* Treats floating wind or wind which is more at the exterior and mobile Usual dosage: 3-10g

Properties when combined:

One treats the lower part of the body, while the other treats the upper part.

When these two medicinals are combined together, they dispel wind, cold, and dampness and treat *bi* over the whole body.

Major indications of the combination:

1. Moving rheumatic pains all over the body (1)
2. Common cold with fever, shivers, headache, back of the neck pain, back pain, and joint pain due to wind, cold, and dampness (2)
3. Joint running wind due to wind, cold, and dampness penetrating the channels and network vessels (3)

Notes:

(1) For these indications, this combination is used in *Juan Bi Tang* (Alleviate Impediment Decoction).

(2) For these indications, this combination is used in *Qiang Huo Sheng Shi Tang* (Notopterygium Overcome Dampness Decoction).

(3) *Li jie feng* or joint running wind refers to acute arthralgia which is severe and movable with loss of joint mobility, swelling, and intense joint pain which is worse at night. This affection can transform itself into heat and then cause redness, pain, swelling, and heat.

Comments:

(a) The ancients did not differentiate between *Du Huo* and *Qiang Huo* since their action is close. They often are clinically combined and, therefore, one frequently sees written in prescriptions: *Er Huo*, the two *Huo*.

(b) *Qiang Huo* has a more powerful action than *Du Huo*. Its nature is upbearing, draining, and vigorous. This is what made the ancients say that *Qiang Huo* has a "masculine dispersing qi."

Du Zhong (Cortex Eucommiae Ulmoidis) & Xu Duan (Radix Dipsaci)

Individual properties:	
Du Zhong	**Xu Duan**
Supplements the liver & kidneys Strengthens sinews & bones Secures the *chong mai* Quiets the fetus Lowers the blood pressure Usual dosage: 10-12g	Supplements the liver & kidneys Strengthens sinews & bones Stops metrorrhagia during pregnancy Quiets the fetus Knits the sinews & bones Usual dosage: 10-12g

Properties when combined:

When these two medicinals are combined together, they mutually reinforce each other. Together, they effectively supplement the liver and kidneys and strengthen the sinews and bones, stop metrorrhagia during pregnancy and quiet the fetus.

Major indications of the combination:

1. Aches and pains, stiffness, lumbar pain, and weakness of lower limbs due to liver-kidney vacuity (1) (4)
2. Knee and lumbar pain due to wind dampness (2)
3. Metrorrhagia during pregnancy and threatened miscarriage accompanied by lumbar pains due to kidney vacuity (1)
4. Traumatic lumbar pain (3) (5)

Notes:

(1) For these indications, salt mix-fried *Du Zhong* and salt mix-fried *Xu Duan* should be prescribed

(2) For these indications, uncooked *Du Zhong* and uncooked *Xu Duan* should be prescribed.

(3) For these indications, wine mix-fried *Xu Duan* and salt mix-fried *Du Zhong* should be prescribed.

(4) For these indications, this combination is used in *Du Zhong Wan* (Eucommia Pills).

(5) For these indications, this combination is included in *Qian Jin Bao Yun Dan* (*Thousand [Pieces of] Gold* Protect Pregnancy Elixir). It is noteworthy that this formula also contains *Bai Zhu* (Rhizoma Atractylodis Macrocephalae) and *Huang Qin* (Radix Scutellariae Baicalensis) which are also key medicinals for quieting the fetus.

Comments:

(a) *Du Zhong* is more powerful than *Xu Duan* to supplement the liver and kidneys, strengthen sinews, bones, and the lumbar area. But *Xu Duan* promotes circulation within the vessels, dispels blood stasis, and knits together fractured bones and torn ligaments.

(b) *Du Zhong* is the major medicinal substance in Chinese medicine for treating lumbar pain. "[For] lumbar pain, one must [use] *Du Zhong*." *Du Zhong* can be used for all types of lumbar pain: vacuity or repletion, hot or cold, if it is combined with other medicinals according to the pattern.

E Jiao (Gelatinum Corii Asini) & *Huang Lian* (Rhizoma Coptidis Chinensis)

Individual properties:	
E Jiao	**Huang Lian**
Nourishes the blood Enriches yin Moistens dryness Stops bleeding Usual dosage: 6-10g	Clears heat and dries dampness Drains fire and resolves toxins Clears & drains heart fire Clears & drains the stomach, liver & intestines Usual dosage: 4-6g

Properties when combined:

One nourishes, while the other clears.
One supplements; the other drains.
When these two medicinals are combined together, they drain fire and enrich yin according to the method of draining the south (*i.e.*, fire) and supplementing the north (*i.e.*, water) and re-establish the interaction between the heart and kidneys. Together, they quiet the spirit and treat dysentery damaging yin.

Major indications of the combination:

1. Vexation and agitation and insomnia due to febrile disease which has damaged yin, vacuity fire, or heart and kidneys not interacting anymore (1) (2)
2. Dysentery which damages yin with pus and blood in the stools due to damp heat in the large intestine (3)

Notes:

(1) For these indications, this combination is present in *Huang Lian E Jiao Tang* (Coptis & Donkey Skin Glue Decoction). For these indications, uncooked *Huang Lian* should be prescribed or, even better, wine-processed *Huang Lian*.

(2) For further discussion of the process of loss of interaction between the heart and kidneys, see the pair *Huang Lian* and *Rou Gui*, note (2) below.

(3) For these indications, uncooked *Huang Lian* should be prescribed.

Comments:

(a) *Huang Lian* is one of the bitterest medicinals in the whole Chinese materia medica. One should be careful not to give too high a dosage of this ingredient to avoid nausea and vomiting which can be caused by this bitterness. In order to avoid this side effect, one can recommend that the patient swallow this decoction while keeping a thin slice of fresh ginger on their tongue or to chew a slice of fresh ginger after swallowing the decoction. Ginger-processing, wine-processing, and stir-frying till yellow are all methods of preparation which tend to alleviate the bitterness of *Huang Lian*.

(b) Many psychological disorders, such as vexation and agitation, loss of memory, insomnia, profuse dreams, and tendency to wake up easily and frequently, are due to loss of interaction between the heart and kidneys. The combination of *E Jiao* and *Huang Lian,* which is present in *Huang Lian E Jiao Tang*, is a key pair for this type of disorder.

(c) *Huang Lian* is incompatible with pork and cold water.

(d) Some treatises say that when *E Jiao* is stored and aged (as in the six aged medicinals; see note (1) of the pair *Ban Xia* and *Chen Pi* above), it is of superior quality. It is then called *Chen E Jiao* (aged *E Jiao*).

(e) *E Jiao* has a remarkable action to promoting red blood cell production and, therefore, treats anemia.

(f) *Chuan Lian*, the Coptis from Sichuan province is believed to be superior to *Yuan Lian*, the Coptis from Yunnan province.

E Zhu (Rhizoma Curcumae Zedoariae) & *San Leng* (Rhizoma Sparganii)

Individual properties:	
E Zhu	**San Leng**
Tropism: liver, spleen & qi division Breaks the qi and quickens the blood (1) Treats qi stagnation which causes blood stasis Treats the blood within the qi Disperses food accumulation Usual dosage: 5-10g	Tropism: liver, spleen & blood division Breaks the blood and moves the qi (1) Treats blood stasis which causes qi stagnation Treats the qi within the blood Usual dosage: 5-10g

Properties when combined:

One is for the qi; the other for the blood. When these two medicinals are combined together, they strongly and effectively break both the qi and blood, regulate and rectify the qi and blood, stop pain and disperse food accumulation.

Major indications of the combination:

1. Abdominal lump glomus, hepatomegaly, and splenomegaly due to blood stasis and/or qi stagnation (2)
2. Amenorrhea, dysmenorrhea, clots in the menstrual flow, and infertility, due to blood stasis (3)
3. Abdominal pain due to food accumulation (4)

Notes:

(1) Readers should note that breaking the qi and

breaking the blood are both attacking methods which can damage the correct qi if used inappropriately, too much, or too long. These treatment methods are more powerful than moving the qi and quickening the blood and should only be used when there is severe qi and blood stasis and stagnation.

(2) For these indications, this combination is found in *E Leng Zhu Yu Tang* (Zedoaria & Sparganium Dispel Stasis Decoction).

(3) For these indications, this combination is found in *San Leng Wan* (Sparganium Pills). For these indications, vinegar mix-fried *E Zhu* and vinegar mix-fried *San Leng* should be prescribed.

(4) For this indication, this combination is present in *E Zhu Wan* (Zedoaria Pills). For these indications, vinegar mix-fried *E Zhu* and uncooked *San Leng* should be prescribed.

Fang Feng (Radix Ledebouriellae Divaricatae) & Huang Qi (Radix Astragali Membranacei)

Individual properties:	
Fang Feng	**Huang Qi**
Acrid, dissipating	Sweet, warm, supplementing
Dispels wind and resolves the exterior	Supplements the qi and upbears yang
Eliminates dampness	Secures the exterior and stops perspiration
Resolves tremors	Disinhibits urination and disperses swelling
Expels external evils	Supports the correct qi
Usual dosage: 6-10g	Usual dosage: 10-20g

Properties when combined:

One dissipates, while the other supplements.
One opens; the other secures.
When these two medicinals are combined together, *Huang Qi* supplements the defensive qi without retaining external evils within the body, while *Fang Feng* drains external evils without damaging correct qi and without causing perspiration. Together, they effectively secure the exterior and supplement the defensive qi, dispel or prevent invasion by external evils and stop perspiration.

Major indications of the combination:

1. Spontaneous perspiration due to exterior vacuity (1)
2. Tendency to catch cold frequently due to defensive qi vacuity (1)

Note:

(1) For these indications, the combination is used in *Yu Ping Feng San* (Jade Windscreen Powder).

Comments:

(a) *Huang Qi* should be prescribed in the form of uncooked *Huang Qi* in order to retain its properties of fluidity and mobility and its tropism towards the exterior. Uncooked *Huang Qi* supplements the defensive qi. This then results in the perfect control of the opening and closing of the pores of the skin and thus a better defense of the exterior against external evils. Uncooked *Fang Feng* (which literally means to prevent or guard against wind) allows the elimination of external evils, namely wind, which penetrate easily through the pores of the skin as soon as they loosen because of a defensive qi weakness.

(b) This combination is present in *Yu Ping Feng San* and is useful to prevent wind attacks. However, it should not be used to treat wind affections which are already established. This combination is too astringent once the evil qi and the defensive qi are already struggling. Its use might, in that case, retain the external evil inside the body. This is likened to shutting all the windows and doors when a thief is inside one's house.

(c) The pair *Fang Feng* and *Huang Qi* when combined with *Zhi Ke* (Fructus Citri Aurantii) gives good results in the treatment of prolapse of the rectum, external hemorrhoids, and flatulence as well as abdominal distention. In terms of rectal prolapse, it is advantageous to add *Fang Feng*, 3g, and *Zhi Ke*, 6g, to *Bu Zhong Yi Qi Tang* (Supplement the Center & Boost the Qi Decoction).

Fu Ling (Sclerotium Poriae Cocos) & Yi Zhi Ren (Fructus Alpiniae Oxyphyllae)

Individual properties:	
Fu Ling	**Yi Zhi Ren**
Fortifies the spleen and supplements the center Percolates dampness and disinhibits urination Tranquilizes the heart and quiets the spirit Supplements and eliminates Usual dosage: 10-15g	Warms the spleen and stops diarrhea Supplements the kidneys and secures the essence Contains the drool and spit and constrains the urine Warms and secures Usual dosage: 6-10g

Properties when combined:

One eliminates; the other secures.
Both supplement.
When these two medicinals are combined together, they complement each other to fortify the spleen, secure the kidneys, reduce urination and stop diarrhea.

Major indications of the combination:

1. Strangury with chyluria, milky, turbid urine, and dysuria due to vacuity cold in the kidneys or kidney qi not securing with imbalance in the function of transformation of the bladder (1)

2. Diarrhea due to vacuity cold of the spleen and kidneys (2)

Notes:

(1) For these indications, salt mix-fried Yi Zhi Ren should be prescribed.

(2) This indication particularly applies to watery diarrhea. Yi Zhi Ren warms the spleen and fortifies the functions of movement and transformation of the spleen, while Fu Ling channels the excess water of the large intestine to the bladder in order to eliminate dampness through urination. For these indications, stir-fried till scorched Yi Zhi Ren should be prescribed.

Fu Xiao Mai (Fructus Levis Tritici Aestivi) & Huang Qi (Radix Astragali Membranacei)

Individual properties:	
Fu Xiao Mai	**Huang Qi**
Sweet, fresh, astringent Supplements the qi and nourishes the heart Clears heat Secures the exterior and stops perspiration Usual dosage: 10-30g	Sweet, warm, supplementing Supplements the qi Repletes the interstices, secures the exterior, and stops perspiration Usual dosage: 10-30g

Properties when combined:

When these two medicinals are combined together, they supplement the qi and nourish the heart, clear heat, secure the exterior, and stop perspiration.

Major indications of the combination:

1. Spontaneous perspiration due to exterior vacuity (1)

Note:

(1) For this indication, this combination is used in *Mu Li San* (Oyster Shell Powder). For this indication, one should prescribe uncooked *Huang Qi* and stir-fried *Fu Xiao Mai*.

Comments:

(a) To treat spontaneous perspiration, *Huang Qi* treats the root (*i.e.*, exterior vacuity), while *Fu Xiao Mai* treats the branch by astringing perspiration.

(b) On the one hand, *Fu Xiao Mai* is light in nature, floating (see comment (c) of the pair *Fu Xiao Ma* and *Ma Huang Gen* below), and is directed at the exterior to stop perspiration. Uncooked *Huang Qi* is light in nature, traveling (as opposed to fixed), and is directed at the exterior and pores of the skin to supplement the defensive qi. These two medicinal substances by their nature and properties have a marked tropism for the exterior. On the other hand, *Xiao Mai* has a heavy nature and honey mix-fried *Huang Qi* has a fixed nature. Therefore, they have a more internal rather than external action.

(c) For further differences between *Fu Xiao Mai* and *Xiao Mai*, see comment (c) of the pair *Fu Xiao Ma* and *Ma Huang Gen* below.

Fu Xiao Mai (Fructus Levis Tritici Aestivi) & *Ma Huang Gen* (Radix Ephedrae)

Individual properties:	
Fu Xiao Mai	**Ma Huang Gen**
Sweet, cool Stops perspiration Tropism: the heart, "Perspiration is the fluid of the heart." Supplements the qi and nourishes the heart Clears heat, stops perspiration, and eliminates vexation Usual dosage: 10-30g	Sweet, neutral Stops perspiration Tropism: the lungs, "The lungs control the skin and are associated with the defensive qi." It is directed to the skin, repletes the exterior, secures the defensive qi, and stops perspiration Usual dosage: 6-10g

Properties when combined:

When these two medicinals are combined together, they effectively supplement the qi and nourish the heart, secure the exterior, clear heat and stop perspiration.

Major indications of the combination:

1. Spontaneous or profuse perspiration due to qi vacuity (1)
2. Night sweats due to vacuity heat or yin vacuity (1)

Note:

(1) For these indications, this combination is used in *Mu Li San* (Oyster Shell Powder).

Comments:

(a) *Fu Xiao Mai* and *Ma Huang Gen* both stop spontaneous perspiration (mainly due to qi vacuity and yang vacuity) or night sweats (mainly due to yin vacuity). However, *Fu Xiao Mai* treats the branch manifestations *and* the root cause (*i.e.*, heart qi vacuity, vacuity heat), while *Ma Huang Gen* only treats the exterior manifestation (*i.e.*, sweating).

(b) It is noteworthy that Ephedra stems (*Ma Huang*) have a diaphoretic effect, while Ephedra roots (*Ma Huang Gen*) and the knots of the Ephedra stem (*Ma Huang Jie*) have an antidiaphoretic action.

(c) Differentiation should be made between *Fu Xiao Mai* and *Xiao Mai*, also called *Huai Xiao Mai*. Both are the grains from the ripe wheat (*Triticum aestivum*), but *Fu Xiao Mai* is the blighted grains which, when dried, float on the surface of the water when wheat is washed, while *Xiao Mai* are the heavy, full grains which sink to the bottom. *Xiao Mai* is superior for nourishing the heart and quieting the spirit, eliminating vexation and treating psychological disorders such as visceral agitation and sadness. *Fu Xiao Mai* is superior for stopping perspiration by astringing, eliminating heat (vacuity), and treating spontaneous perspiration, night sweats, or the feeling of heat in the bones. In addition, stir-fried *Fu Xiao Mai* is more powerful than uncooked *Fu Xiao Mai* for stopping sweating. In terms of *Xiao Mai*, the wheat from southern China is reputed to be warm, while that from the north is believed to be cool. *Chen Xiao Mai* is wheat which has been stored and aged. This is preferred by some practitioners, since the more recent wheat, freshly harvested, is too warm in nature. This warmth is lost when aged. *Bai Mian* is wheat flour. When stir-fried (*Chao Mian*), it supplements the spleen and stops diarrhea.

Fu Zi (Radix Lateralis Praeparatus Aconiti Carmichaeli) & *Gan Jiang* (Dry Rhizoma Zingiberis)

Individual properties:	
Fu Zi	**Gan Jiang**
Acrid, very hot Mobile Quickens the yang in the 12 channels In the exterior, it is directed to the skin to drain cold. In the interior, it is directed to the three burners to drain cold. Makes the yang return and relieves from counterflow Usual dosage: 6-10g	Acrid, hot Fixed Warms the spleen & stomach and drains cold Warms the lungs and transforms phlegm cold Reinforces *Fu Zi* Makes yang return and relieves from counterflow Usual dosage: 6-10g

Properties when combined:

When these two medicinals are combined together, they effectively reinforce each other, return yang, and stem counterflow.

Major indications of the combination:

1. Loss of consciousness, cold spontaneous perspiration, cold limbs, and a minute pulse due to yang desertion (1)
2. Pain and a feeling of cold in the stomach and abdomen, vomiting, and diarrhea due to spleen vacuity cold (2)

Notes:

(1) For these indications, this combination is used in *Si Ni Tang* (Four Counterflows Decoction). For these indications, bland *Fu Zi* should be prescribed

(2) For these indications, this combination is present in *Fu Zi Li Zhong Wan* (Aconite Rectify the Center Pills). For these indications, blast-fried *Fu Zi* should be prescribed

Comments:

(a) *Gan Jiang* is inferior to Fu Zi for returning yang and stemming counterflow. However, these two substances are very often combined to treat this type of problem because *Gan Jiang* reinforces the action of *Fu Zi*. This is illustrated by the saying, "*Fu Zi* without *Gan Jiang* is not warm."

(b) It is stated above that, "In the interior, *Fu Zi* is directed towards the three burners in order to drain cold." This means that *Fu Zi* has a general action over the whole body. In fact, it invigorates life gate fire, assists original yang, and thus acts mainly on heart yang (upper burner), spleen yang (middle burner), and kidney yang (lower burner).

(c) For precautions when using *Fu Zi*, see comment (b) of the pair *Da Huang* and *Fu Zi* above.

Fu Zi (Radix Lateralis Praeparatus Aconiti Carmichaeli) & *Huang Qi* (Radix Astragali Membranacei)

Individual properties:	
Fu Zi	*Huang Qi*
Returns yang and stems counterflow	Supplements the qi and upbears yang
Warms the kidneys and invigorates yang	Secures the exterior and stops perspiration
Drains cold and stops pain	Disinhibits urination and disperses swelling
Strongly supplements yang	Strongly supplements the qi
Treats collapse	Treats perspiration
Usual dosage: 6-10g	Usual dosage: 10-30g

Properties when combined:

One is for yang, while the other is for the qi. One is for collapse; the other for perspiration. When these two medicinals are combined together, they complement and reinforce each other. Together, they effectively supplement the qi and warm yang, return yang, secure the exterior, and stop perspiration.

Major indications of the combination:

1. Cold spontaneous perspiration accompanied by fear of cold, cold limbs, lassitude of the spirit, a pale tongue with white fur, and a fine, weak pulse, and in severe cases, profuse perspiration, loss of consciousness, and a minute pulse due to yang vacuity or yang collapse (1)

Note:

(1) For these indications, bland *Fu Zi* and uncooked *Huang Qi* should be prescribed.

Gan Cao (Radix Glycyrrhizae) & *Hua Shi* (Talcum)

Individual properties:	
Gan Cao	**Hua Shi**
Harmonizing Drains fire Resolves toxins Moderates the cold nature of *Hua Shi* and protects the middle burner Usual dosage: 3- 6g	Slippery in nature, disinhibiting (1) Above, it clears the origin of water, *i.e.*, the lungs, and downbears the lung qi. Below, it frees the flow of the water passageways and opens the bladder. Eliminates evil heat in the six bowels Drains summerheat and eliminates vexation Prevents stasis due to the sweet flavor of *Gan Cao* Usual dosage: 10-18g

Properties when combined:

When these two medicinals are combined together, they clear heat, eliminate summerheat, and disinhibit urination without damaging the middle burner. Together, they disinhibit urination and free strangury.

Major indications of the combination:

1. Fever, vexation and agitation, thirst, vomiting, diarrhea, and dysuria due to attack of summerheat with internal and external heat (2)
2. Turbid strangury
3. Stone and/or sand strangury

Notes:

(1) Literally, *Hua Shi* means slippery stone or the stone which causes slipping. This substance takes its name from the fact that, when powdered, it is slippery to the touch. It is also a mineral which allows a "sliding" movement to sand strangury. Furthermore, some prescriptions use it to "make the fetus slide" in order to hasten delivery.

(2) For these indications, this combination is used in *Liu Yi San* (Six to One Powder).

Comments:

(a) *Hua Shi* is cold and, therefore, clears heat. It is bland and, therefore, disinhibits urination. It is heavy (being a mineral) and, therefore, favors descent. It is slippery and, therefore, frees the portals or orifices. These are the reasons why the use of *Hua Shi* is not advisable during pregnancy. In that case, it might cause the fetus to slide. Note, for instance, that repeated miscarriage in Chinese medicine is called slippery fetus.

(b) For all these indications, *Gan Cao Shao* (Extremitas Radicis Glycyrrhizae) is superior to *Gan Cao* for disinhibiting urination and freeing strangury.

(c) *Gan Cao* is incompatible with pork, seaweed (particularly *Hai Zao* [Herba Sargassii]), and Chinese cabbage (*Brassica Chinensis* or *Brassica Pekinensis*).

Gan Cao (Radix Glycyrrhizae) & *Jie Geng* (Radix Platycodi Grandiflori)

Individual properties:	
Gan Cao	***Jie Geng***
Sweet, harmonizing, cool	Acrid and dissipating, bitter and draining
Clears heat and resolves toxins	Diffuses and frees the flow of the lung qi
Moistens the lungs	Disinhibits the throat
Transforms phlegm	Transforms phlegm
Relieves tension and stops pain	Evacuates pus
Harmonizes other medicinal substances and	Guides other medicinal substances towards the
protects the middle burner	upper part of the body and towards the lungs
Usual dosage: 5-10g	Usual dosage: 9-15g

Properties when combined:

One clears, while the other diffuses.
One moderates; the other drains.
When these two medicinals are combined together, they effectively clear heat and transform phlegm, disinhibit the throat and stop pain, evacuate pus and resolve toxins.

Major indications of the combination:

1. Pulmonary abscess with cough, expectoration of profuse, purulent phlegm, and chest oppression and pain due to heat stasis in the chest (1)
2. Pain, redness, and swelling of the throat due to heat (vacuity or repletion, external or internal) (2)
3. Loss of voice and/or hoarse or husky voice (2)

Notes:

(1) For these indications, this combination is present in *Jie Geng Tang* (Platycodon Decoction).

(2) For these indications, this combination can be reinforced by *He Zi* (Fructus Terminaliae Chebulae) as in *He Zi Tang* (Terminalia Decoction). For these indications, in case of lung dryness, honey mix-fried *Jie Geng* should be prescribed. For phlegm dampness, use uncooked *Jie Geng*.

Comments:

(a) *Jie Geng* is a key medicinal substance for lung disorders, such as cough, chest oppression, chest pain, sore throat, aphonia, and bronchial phlegm. It can be prescribed for all sorts of pain in the throat or cough accompanied by phlegm when combined with other medicinals appropriate for the pattern.

(b) *Jie Geng* is a messenger remedy (literally, a boat remedy) which guides the action of other medicinal substances towards the lungs and chest or the hand *tai yin* channel. Thus *Jie Geng* can raise medicinals which otherwise have a tropism for the lower burner towards the middle or upper burner.

(c) *Jie Geng* can be used to treat certain types of oliguria, anuria, and dysuria (*i.e.*, disorders of the lower part of the body) by stimulating the superior origin of fluids — the lungs. This is an example of the principle of treating diseases in the lower body by acting on the upper body. "(When) a disease is located in the lower [part], choose the upper [part]."

(d) *Jie Geng* is incompatible with pork. *Gan Cao* is incompatible with pork, seaweed, and Chinese cabbage.

Gan Jiang (Dry Rhizoma Zingiberis) & Huang Lian (Rhizoma Coptidis Chinensis)

Individual properties:	
Gan Jiang	**Huang Lian**
Acrid, warm, frees the flow and opens	Bitter, cold, downbearing, draining
Warms the middle burner and drains cold	Clears heat and dries dampness
Returns yang and frees the flow of the channels	Drains fire and resolves toxins
Treats diarrhea and vomiting due to cold	Treats diarrhea and vomiting due to heat
Usual dosage: 3-10g (1)	Usual dosage: 3-10g (1)

Properties when combined:

One is acrid and frees the flow, while the other is bitter and drains.

One is warm and dissipating; the other is cold and downbearing.

One supplements spleen yang; the other clears replete heat.

When these two medicinals are combined together, they eliminate cold accumulation and depressive heat. Together, they effectively drain mixed cold and heat in order to stop vomiting and diarrhea.

Major indications of the combination:

1. Vomiting, acid regurgitation, belching, epigastric pain or distention, and clamoring stomach (2) due to a mixture of heat and cold in the stomach (3) (4)
2. Diarrhea, dysentery, and stomach rumbling due to mixed heat and cold and/or disharmony between the stomach and intestines (4)
3. Glossitis, stomatitis, and chronic, recalcitrant mouth ulcers due to spleen yang vacuity and stomach fire

Notes:

(1) In case of predominant heat, one can prescribe a small quantity of Gan Jiang and a larger quantity of Huang Lian. In case of predominant cold, one can prescribe a small quantity of Huang Lian and a larger quantity of Gan Jiang. If cold and heat are in equal proportion, an equal quantity of Huang Lian and Gan Jiang should be prescribed.

(2) Clamoring stomach refers to a feeling of hunger, burning, emptiness, unease, and sometimes pain in the stomach with nausea and acid regurgitation.

(3) For these indications, this combination is included in Ban Xia Xie Xin Tang (Pinellia Drain the Heart Decoction).

(4) For these indications, stir-fried Huang Lian should be prescribed unless heat is severe, in which case, uncooked Huang Lian should be prescribed.

Comment:

Heat fights cold, and cold fights heat. The acrid taste quickens, frees the flow, and upbears. The bitter taste drains and downbears. The combination of Gan Jiang (hot, acrid) and Huang Lian (cold, bitter) allows one to regulate upbearing and downbearing, to harmonize yin and yang, and to treat mixed cold and heat which provokes epigastric distention, nausea, vomiting, rumbling, diarrhea, etc.

Gan Jiang (Dry Rhizoma Zingiberis) & Wu Wei Zi (Fructus Schisandrae Chinensis)

Individual properties:	
Gan Jiang	*Wu Wei Zi*
Acrid, dissipating, warm, frees the flow Warms the spleen and drains cold Warms the lungs and transforms phlegm Usual dosage: 6-10g	Sour, astringent Secures the lung qi Stops coughs and calms asthma Usual dosage: 3-10g

Properties when combined:

One drains; the other secures.
One frees the flow; the other astringes.
One treats the root; the other treats the branch.
When these two medicinals are combined together, they mutually complement each other. Together, they effectively warm the lungs and transform phlegm, stop cough and calm asthma.

Major indications of the combination:

1. Cough and/or asthma accompanied by profuse, clear, and white phlegm due to cold in the lungs, lung yang vacuity, or phlegm cold (1)

Note:

(1) For these indications, this combination is used in *Xiao Qing Long Tang* (Minor Blue Dragon Decoction) accompanied by *Xi Xin* (Herba Asari Cum Radice).

Comments:

(a) On the one hand, *Gan Jiang* warms the spleen and stimulates its functions of transformation and transportation. This has the effect of promoting the upbearing of the clear towards the lungs and the downbearing of the turbid towards the large intestine. Furthermore, it prevents the engenderment of phlegm which the spleen tends to discharge into the lungs. On the other hand, *Gan Jiang* transforms accumulated cold phlegm in the lungs by warming the lungs, remembering that the Chinese word for transform also means to melt. This then promotes diffusion and downbearing. In turn, this has the effect of regulating and freeing the flow of the water passageways in order to prevent the engenderment of new phlegm and downbearing the counterflowing lung qi. While *Gan Jiang* treats the disease mechanism or root of the disease, *Wu Wei Zi* treats the branch manifestations, *i.e.*, cough and asthma, by securing the lung qi due to its astringent nature. For more details on the effects of *Wu Wei Zi* in the treatment of coughs and asthma, see comment (a) in the pair *Wu Wei Zi* and *Xi Xin* below.

(b) In clinical practice, *Gan Jiang* has clearly demonstrated its efficacy for cold type asthma. It is, therefore, often systematically added to reinforce the impact of conventional treatments for this pattern of cough and asthma.

Gao Liang Jiang (Rhizoma Alpiniae Officinari) & *Xiang Fu* (Rhizoma Cyperi Rotundi)

Individual properties:	
Gao Liang Jiang	**Xiang Fu**
Warms the stomach Scatters cold Stops pain & vomiting Usual dosage: 6-10g	Drains the liver Moves the qi Stops pain Usual dosage: 6-10g

Properties when combined:

One warms, while the other moves. When these two medicinals are combined together, they effectively warm the stomach and drain cold, move the qi and stop pain.

Major indications of the combination:

1. Pain in the epigastrium alleviated by warmth and pressure, chest and lateral costal distention, and nausea due to cold in the stomach and qi stagnation (1)

Note:

(1) For these indications, this combination is used in *Liang Fu Wan* (Galangal & Cyperus Pills). For these indications, vinegar mix-fried *Xiang Fu* should be prescribed.

Comments:

(a) In case of severe cold, a greater quantity of *Gao Liang Jiang* should be prescribed. In case of severe qi stagnation, as evidenced by epigastric distention and pain aggravated by pressure, a greater quantity of *Xiang Fu* should be prescribed.

(b) *Gao Liang Jiang* is very acrid and drying. Its action is drastic, and it should not be prescribed over a long period of time for fear of damaging stomach qi and yin.

Ge Gen (Radix Puerariae) & *Sheng Ma* (Rhizoma Cimicifugae)

Individual properties:	
Ge Gen	**Sheng Ma**
Resolves the muscle aspect Eliminates heat Out-thrusts rashes Engenders fluids and stops thirst Tends to reach evils horizontally and, therefore, out-thrusts rashes on the back and middle part of the body Usual dosage: 6-10g	Resolves the exterior Clears heat Out-thrusts rashes Upbears yang qi Tends to be upbearing, raising and reaching evils in the upper part of the body and, therefore, out-thrusts eruptions on the neck and face Usual dosage: 3-6g

Properties when combined:

When these two medicinals are combined together, they resolve the exterior and muscle aspect, clear heat and resolve toxins, and out-thrust rashes in the whole body.

Major indications for the combination:

1. Skin rashes which have difficulty coming out accompanied by headache and fever due to an exterior pattern (1) (3)

2. Measles in the initial stage (1) with eruptions which have difficulty coming out and fever sometimes accompanied by lack of perspiration or perspiration which has difficulty in coming out (2) due to an exterior pattern (3)

Notes:

(1) For these indications, this combination is used in *Sheng Ma Ge Gen Tang* (Cimicifuga & Pueraria Decoction).

(2) For these indications, this combination is present in *Xuan Du Jie Biao Tang* (Diffuse Toxins & Resolve the Exterior Decoction).

(3) For all of these indications, uncooked *Ge Gen* and uncooked *Sheng Ma* should be prescribed.

Comments:

(a) *Ge Gen* and *Sheng Ma* both upbear yang. However, *Sheng Ma* is more powerful than *Ge Gen*. Moreover, *Sheng Ma* is used for all types of qi fall in the middle burner, such as ptosis of the organs, rectal prolapse, prolapse of the uterus, shortness of breath with a feeling of collapse in the chest, chronic diarrhea, and persistent metrorrhagia, while *Ge Gen* is only used for diarrhea. It treats diarrhea of either the vacuity type (*i.e.*, spleen vacuity) or repletion type (*i.e.*, damp heat). For these indications, roasted *Ge Gen* should be prescribed.

(b) *Sheng Ma* is a messenger medicinal which guides the action of other medicinal substances towards the upper part of the body — the head, face, and upper orifices — and towards the *yang ming*. Therefore, it is used to treat toothache, oral ulcers, and stomatitis associated with the stomach and constipation associated with the large intestine.

(c) *Ge Gen* has numerous interesting modern applications. For instance, it is used to treat high blood pressure, hypercholesterolemia, coronary disease, angina pectoris, headaches and painful tension in the cervical area due to high blood pressure, and sudden deafness. These uses are based on this medicinal's marked effect of dilating the blood vessels.

Gou Qi Zi (Fructus Lycii Chinensis) & *Ju Hua* (Flos Chrysanthemi Morifolii)

Individual properties:	
Gou Qi Zi	*Ju Hua*
Nourishing & moistening in nature Supplements the kidneys and fills the essence Nourishes liver blood and brightens the eyes Usual dosage: 10-15g	Light & upbearing in nature Dispels wind and clears heat Calms the liver and brightens the eyes Usual dosage: 10-15g

Properties when combined:

One nourishes, while the other brightens.
One supplements; the other calms.
When these two medicinals are combined together, they effectively nourish and supplement the liver and kidneys, clear heat and calm the liver, and brighten the eyes.

Major indications of the combination:

1. Blurred vision, diminished visual acuity, "moving black spots in front of the eyes", fire sparks in the eyes, photophobia, dry eyes with distention and headache, and pain in the lower back and knees due to liver-kidney vacuity (1) (2) (3)

Notes:

(1) For these indications, this combination is present in *Qi Ju Di Huang Wan* (Lycium & Chrysanthemum Rehmannia Pills).

(2) For these indications, *Bai Ju Hua* (white *Ju Hua*) should be prescribed. See comment (a) of the pair *Ju Hua* and *Sang Ye* below.

(3) The ascending property and tropism of *Ju Hua* being towards the liver and eyes, carries the action of *Gou Qi Zi* towards the eyes.

Comments:

(a) Although the usual dosage of *Ju Hua* is 10-15g per day, for eye problems, headaches with a feeling of distention, or hypertension, a greater quantity of *Ju Hua* (20-30g) must be used to benefit from its therapeutic action.

(b) In case of loose stools or diarrhea due to qi vacuity or spleen yang vacuity, it is worthwhile to prescribe stir-fried *Gou Qi Zi* in order to lessen its slightly cold and moistening nature which tends to damage the spleen. However, when prepared in this way, *Gou Qi Zi* tends to nourish the blood and essence, the liver and kidneys less strongly.

(c) (*Bai*) *Ju Hua* gives very good results in hypertensive disorders, especially when accompanied by vertigo and headaches mainly due to liver yang rising. It is often combined with *Shan Zha* (Fructus Crataegi), 15-20g per day, in case of hypercholesterolemia.

Gua Lou (Fructus Trichosanthis Kirlowii) & *Xie Bai* (Bulbus Allii)

Individual properties:	
Gua Lou	**Xie Bai**
Sweet and cold, moistening, clearing, downbearing	Acrid and warm, frees the flow, dissipating, moving
Clears the lungs	Warms the chest and frees the flow of yang
Transforms phlegm	Opens the portals of the heart
Loosens the chest and scatters nodulations	Moves the qi and scatters nodulation
Moistens dryness and moistens the intestines	Quickens the blood and stops pain
Loosens the chest & diaphragm and frees the flow of impediment	Treats chest *bi* and yin binding or qi stagnation constipation
Usual dosage: 10-20g	Usual dosage: 5-15g

Properties when combined:

One moistens, while the other dissipates.
One loosens; the other frees the flow.
When these two medicinals are combined together, they effectively free the flow of yang and move the qi, loosen the chest and clear the lungs, transform phlegm and scatter nodulation, stop pain, and moisten the intestines and free the flow of the stools.

Major indications of the combination:

1. Constipation due to fluid dryness of the large intestine and/or to qi stagnation (4)
2. Yin binding constipation (1) (4)
3. Chest *bi* with oppression of the chest and epigastrium, cough, profuse phlegm, piercing pain in the chest radiating towards the back, and shortness of breath due to accumulation of turbid phlegm blocking the qi and yang of the chest (2)(5)

4. Chest *bi* and cardiac disease with intense heart pain due to heart qi and blood stasis and stagnation and deficiency of chest yang (3) (5)

Notes:

(1) Yin binding constipation refers to constipation due to spleen-kidney yang vacuity or sometimes due to dryness in the large intestine caused by an essence blood deficiency with pale lips, white tongue fur, and clear, long urination.

(2) For these indications, this combination is used in *Gua Lou Xie Bai Ban Xia Tang* (Trichosanthes, Allium & Pinellia Decoction) which can be favorably combined with *Er Chen Tang* (Two Aged [Ingredients] Decoction).

(3) For these indications, this combination is included in *Gua Lou Xie Bai Bai Jiu Tang* (Trichosanthes, Allium & White Alcohol Decoction) and it can be favorably reinforced by *Dan Shen* (Radix Salviae Miltiorrhizae), *San Qi* (Radix Pseudoginseng), *Tan Xiang* (Lignum Santali Albi), and *Gui Zhi* (Ramulus Cinnamomi Cassiae).

(4) For these indications, one should prescribe uncooked *Gua Lou*. See note (c) below.

(5) For these indications, one should prescribe stir-fried till scorched *Gua Lou*. Also see note (c) below.

Comments:

(a) *Gua Lou* is sweet and cold. However, it is used for chest *bi* due to qi stagnation and blood stasis and/or to chest yang vacuity. In fact, *Gua Lou* is sweet, but it does not supplement nor produce qi stagnation. *Gua Lou* is cold but does not cause obstruction. On the contrary, *Gua Lou* tends to promote circulation of qi, to expel phlegm, to loosen the chest, and to scatter nodulation. Furthermore, in case of chest yang vacuity or stasis and stagnation, *Gua Lou* is combined with medicinal substances that balance its cold nature, such as *Xie Bai* (Bulbus Allii), *Bai Jiu* (white alcohol), *Gui Zhi* (Ramulus Cinnamomi Cassiae), and *Tan Xiang* (Lignum Santali Albi).

(b) There are several medicinals derived from the Trichosanthes plant. *Gua Lou Gen* or *Tian Hua Fen* is Radix Trichosanthis Kirlowii, the plant's root. *Gua Lou Pi* is Pericarpium Trichosanthis Kirlowii, the skin of the fruit. *Gua Lou Ren* is Semen Trichosanthis Kirlowii, the seed from the fruit. *Gua Lou* or *Quan Gua Lou* is Fructus Trichosanthis Kirlowii, the entire fruit with the skin and the seeds. *Gua Lou Ren* moistens the intestines, frees the flow of the stools, and, therefore, treats constipation. *Gua Lou Pi* clears the lungs and transforms phlegm, loosens the chest and treats chest *bi*. *Quan Gua Lou* includes all the functions and indications of *Gua Lou Ren* and *Gua Lou Pi*. However, *Gua Lou Pi* is more efficient than *Quan Gua Lou* for treating chest *bi*. While *Gua Lou Ren* is more efficient than *Quan Gua Lou* for treating constipation. It is for these reasons that it is advised to use *Gua Lou Ren* in case of constipation and *Gua Lou Pi* in case of chest *bi*.

(c) Modern research has demonstrated that *Xie Bai* (Herba Allii) lowers serum cholesterol.

Gui Zhi (Ramulus Cinnamomi Cassiae) & Ma Huang (Herba Ephedrae)

Individual properties:	
Gui Zhi	**Ma Huang**
Directed towards the heart channel and the blood (& constructive) division Acrid, sweet, warm Dispels evils and harmonizes the constructive qi Resolves the muscles and dispels wind evils (moderate diaphoretic) Usual dosage: 6-10g	Directed towards the lung channel and the qi (& defensive) division Acrid, bitter Opens the interstices and scatters cold evils Effuses sweat and scatters cold (powerful diaphoretic) Usual dosage: 3-10g

Properties when combined:

When these two medicinals are combined together, they act to mutually reinforce each other's floating and dispelling characteristics. Together, they effectively open the pores of the skin, strongly provoke perspiration, resolve the muscles, and scatter wind cold of the replete type.

Major indications of the combination:

1. Colds, influenza with fever, fear of cold, severe shivering, absence of perspiration, headache, and general body aches caused by wind cold of the replete type
2. Rheumatic pains due to wind, cold, and dampness (1)
3. Cough and asthma due to wind cold obstructing the lung qi (1)

Note:

(1) For this indication, this combination is found in Ma Huang Tang (Ephedra Decoction). For this indication, uncooked Gui Zhi and uncooked Ma Huang should be prescribed. However, it is advisable to use honey mix-fried Ma Huang for cough and asthma.

Comments:

(a) In winter, cold is exuberant. By its nature, it congeals and contracts. When it attacks the body, it creates first an obstacle to the lung qi and exterior qi (i.e., mainly the defensive qi). Moreover, winter is the season of introversion, of storage, of interiorization. Fluids are deeply concealed in the system. Therefore, a powerful action is required to mobilize these fluids and bring them to the exterior in order to cause perspiration which will free the lungs and the exterior. Gui Zhi communicates with the constructive division where it moves fluids. It brings these fluids to the exterior where Ma Huang then pushes them outward forcefully in order to eliminate external cold. The complementarity of these two medicinals is well illustrated by the saying, "Gui Zhi is not as good as Ma Huang, (but) Ma Huang is not good without Gui Zhi."

(b) Ma Huang is a sudorific, while the root of Ephedra (Ma Huang Gen) and the knots of the stem of Ephedra (Ma Huang Jie) are antisudorific. This is why the original text of the Shang Han Lun (Treatise on Cold Damage) advises for Ma Huang Tang (Ephedra Decoction), which aims at causing perspiration, to use Ma Huang without the knots of the stem in order to make its sudorific effect powerful.

(c) Ma Huang is a very active and powerful substance whose use requires some precautions. It is strongly contraindicated to use Ma Huang in too large a dose (more than 10g per day) and over a long period of time. Its draining action tends to damage qi and yin. Traditionally, Ma Huang must be cooked before the other medicinals in order to eliminate the foam caused by cooking before continuing to decoct the other medicinals. According to ancient authors, this foam contains a large quantity of the active substances which give *Ma Huang* its drastic power to cause perspiration and calm asthma. Ingesting this foam, or rather the substances which it contains, can cause vexation and agitation and even heart palpitations and hypertension. Eliminating this foam allows one to alleviate this drastic action of *Ma Huang* and, therefore, lessen its secondary effects. Nevertheless, nowadays in China, for practical reasons, this foam is not eliminated, and *Ma Huang* is cooked at the end of the decoction for five minutes with the other medicinals. Secondary effects can be controlled by reducing the dosage of *Ma Huang* and its length of administration.

(d) *Gui Zhi* and *Ma Huang* have a similar action. These two medicinals, acrid and warm, facilitate perspiration, resolve the exterior, and are often combined to powerfully induce perspiration in order to treat wind cold attacks. In addition, *Gui Zhi* and *Ma Huang* induce diuresis and treat edema. Nevertheless, one must differentiate their mode of functioning to be able to prescribe them correctly.

Gui Zhi is a moderate sudorific. It treats wind cold of the vacuity type with disharmony between the constructive and defensive and spontaneous perspiration. For this, it is combined with *Bai Shao* (Radix Albus Paeoniae Lactiflorae). *Ma Huang* is a powerful sudorific. It treats wind cold of the replete type with absence of perspiration. For this, it is combined with *Gui Zhi*. *Gui Zhi* warms and frees the flow of yang and promotes urination by stimulating the function of transformation of the bladder. It treats edema from below. It treats edema of the damp type due to deficiency of the transformative function of the bladder. *Ma Huang* diffuses the lung qi and promotes diuresis by stimulating the upper source of fluids (*i.e.*, the lungs). In other words, it drains and downbears the lung qi, thus treating edema from above. *Ma Huang* treats the wind type of edema due to a blockage of the lung qi by external wind.

Gui Zhi (Ramulus Cinnamomi Cassiae) & *Shi Gao* (Gypsum Fibrosum)

Individual properties:	
Gui Zhi	**Shi Gao**
Warm, acrid, dissipating, moving Directed towards the blood division Resolves the muscles and expels wind Warms the channels and quickens the network vessels Usual dosage: 6-10g	Very cold, acrid, clearing, draining Directed towards the qi division Clears heat from the muscles & internal heat Usual dosage: 20-30g

Properties when combined:

One is warm, while the other is very cold.
One moves; the other clears.
Both are acrid.
When these two medicinals are combined together, they clear heat and free the flow of the network vessels, stop pain and treat heat *bi* or impediment.

Major indications of the combination:

1. Rheumatic pain of the heat type with redness, heat, swelling and severe pain in the joints (1)

Note:

(1) For this indication, this combination is used in *Bai Hu Gui Zhi Tang* (White Tiger & Cinnamon Twig Decoction). For this indication, uncooked *Gui Zhi* and uncooked *Shi Gao* should be prescribed.

Comments:

(a) *Gui Zhi Mu*, *i.e.*, the small twigs of Cinnamon from which the external bark has been removed, is less powerful than *Gui Zhi* for resolving the exterior and inducing perspiration but is more powerful for warming the channels and quickening the network vessels. This is why *Gui Zhi Mu* is preferred for the treatment of joint pain and stiffness of the sinews.

(b) To treat inflammatory rheumatism or heat *bi*, *Shi Gao* should be prescribed up to 150g per day and, in severe cases, up to 250g per day.

(c) To facilitate the extraction of the active principles of *Shi Gao* in decoction, it is advised to use *Shi Gao* in powder form and to cook it 30 minutes before adding the other ingredients.

Hai Jin Sha (Spora Lygodii) & Ji Nei Jin (Endothelium Corneum Gigeriae Galli)

Individual properties:	
Hai Jin Sha	*Ji Nei Jin*
Disinhibits urination Frees strangury Drains damp heat Usual dosage: 10-15g	Softens, transforms, and disperses stones Frees strangury Disperses food stagnation Usual dosage: 5-10g

Properties when combined:

One drains, while the other transforms. When these two medicinals are combined together, they free strangury, transform stones, and, therefore, treat stone strangury.

Major indications of the combination:

1. Stone strangury and urinary lithiasis due to damp heat

Comments:

(a) This combination can be advantageously reinforced by combining it with *Ji Qian Cao* (Herba Desmodii Seu Lysimachiae), *Hua Shi* (Talcum), *Qu Mai* (Herba Dianthi), and *Che Qian Zi* (Semen Plantaginis).

(b) *Ji Nei Jin* may also be used for gallstones.

Hai Jin Sha (Spora Lygodii) & Jin Qian Cao (Herba Desmodii Seu Lysimachiae)

Individual properties:	
Hai Jin Sha	*Jin Qian Cao*
Clears heat from the small intestine, bladder & blood division Disinhibits urination Frees strangury Usual dosage: 10-15g	Clears heat and eliminates dampness Disinhibits the gallbladder and treats jaundice Disinhibits urination and frees strangury Expels stones and stops pain Usual dosage: 10-30g

Properties when combined:

When these two medicinals are combined together, they complement and mutually reinforce each other. Together, they strongly clear heat and eliminate dampness, disinhibit urination and free strangury, and expel stones.

Major indications of the combination:

1. Stone and/or sand strangury, renal lithiasis, bladder lithiasis (1)
2. Gallstones due to damp heat in the gallbladder (2)

Notes:

(1) For these indications, this combination can be advantageously reinforced by combining it with *Ji Nei Jin* (Endothelium Corneum Gigeriae Galli), *Che Qian Zi* (Semen Plantaginis), *Dong Gua Ren* (Semen Benincasae Hispidae), and *Qu Mai* (Herba Dianthi).

(2) For these indications, this combination can be advantageously reinforced by combining it with *Yin Chen Hao* (Herba Artemisiae Capillaris), *Yu Jin* (Tuber Curcumae), *Jiang Huang* (Rhizoma Curcumae Longae), *Qing Pi* (Pericarpium Citri Reticulatae Viride), and *Hu Zhang* (Radix Et Rhizoma Polygoni Cuspidati).

Comment:

(a) *Jin Qian Cao* is very effective in cases of biliary or renal lithiasis (*i.e.*, stone and/or sand strangury) and may be used all by itself. In that case, 200-250g of *Jin Qian Cao* should be prescribed. In cases where *Jin Qian Cao* is combined with other medicinals, a relatively high dosage should still be maintained: 50-150g/day.

Hai Tong Pi (Cortex Erythriniae) & *Qin Jiao* (Radix Gentianae Macrophyllae)

Individual properties:	
Hai Tong Pi	***Qin Jiao***
Dispels wind and eliminates dampness Frees the flow of the network vessels and stops pain Clears & eliminates dampness & heat A bark, it treats pain in the upper part of the body. Usual dosage: 6-10g	Dispels wind Frees the flow of the network vessels Soothes the sinews and frees the flow of the channels A root, it treats pain in the lower part of the body. Usual dosage: 6-12g

Properties when combined:

One treats the upper, while the other treats the lower.
When these two medicinals are combined together, they free the flow and quicken the 12 channels in the upper and lower parts of the body, dispel wind dampness and stop pain.

Major indications of the combination:

1. Myalgia in the whole body, lumbar pain, pain in the legs, joint pain, and cramps due to wind dampness or wind, dampness, and heat which produces impediment of the qi in the channels (1)
2. The sequelae of infantile paralysis

Note:

(1) This combination treats *bi* due to heat or wind, dampness, and heat. In that case, it may be favorably reinforced by combining it with *Sang Zhi* (Ramulus Mori Albi), *Ren Dong Teng* (Caulis Lonicerae Japonicae), and *Hong Teng* (Caulis Sargentodoxae).

Han Fang Ji (Radix Stephaniae Tetrandrae) & Huang Qi (Radix Astragali Membranacei)

Individual properties:	
Han Fang Ji	**Huang Qi**
Bitter, cold, downbearing, draining Quickens the channels Opens the pores of the skin Opens the nine portals or orifices Disinhibits urination and disperses swelling Dispels wind dampness and stops pain Drains evil qi Usual dosage: 6-10g	Sweet, warm, upbearing, supplementing Supplements the middle burner and upbears yang Secures the exterior and stops perspiration Supplements the qi and disinhibits urination Promotes diuresis and disperses swelling Promotes tissue regeneration Supplements the correct qi Usual dosage: 10-15g

Properties when combined:

One drains, the other supplements.
When these two medicinals are combined together, they simultaneously drain and supplement. They support the correct qi and drain evil qi at the same time.
One downbears; the other upbears.
Together, they regulate the upbearing and downbearing of the qi mechanism and strongly promote diuresis.

Major indications of the combination:

1. Edema due to wind water with fever, fear of wind, edema predominantly in the upper body and face, joint pain, scanty urination, and a floating pulse (1) (2)
2. Rheumatic pain due to damp *bi* with heavy limbs, joint numbness, and sometimes swollen joints (1) (3)
3. Chronic nephritis and cardiac disease with edema due to qi vacuity and accumulation of dampness (1)

Notes:

(1) For these indications, this combination is found in *Fang Ji Huang Qi Tang* (Stephania & Astragalus Decoction).

(2) If wind attacks the exterior and blocks the

lung qi, this causes a disturbance in the lungs' diffusing and downbearing function. Therefore, because the water passageways are not regulated, dampness is not moved downward. Thus there is accumulation of dampness in the upper body and edema appears.

(3) For edema and oliguria, *Han Fang Ji* (Radix Stephaniae Tetrandrae) is superior. For rheumatic complaints due to wind dampness, *Mu Fang Ji* (Radix Cocculi) is superior. *Han Fang Ji* tends to treat lower body edema. *Mu Fang Ji* tends to treat upper body edema.

Comments:

(a) For all these indications, uncooked *Huang Qi* should be prescribed.

(b) In *Fang Ji Huang Qi Tang*, *Fang Ji*, *Huang Qi*, and *Bai Zhu* (Rhizoma Atractylodis Macrocephalae) promote diuresis and treat edema. *Han Fan Ji* promotes diuresis essentially by draining the bladder. *Huang Qi* promotes diuresis essentially by supplementing the lung qi which is the upper origin of the water passageways and which diffuses and downbears fluids. *Bai Zhu* promotes diuresis by fortifying the spleen qi to transform dampness.

(c) Usually, *Han Fang Ji* is known for its treatment of edema in the lower half of the body and accumulation of damp heat in the lower burner. When combined with *Huang Qi* (which is moving and light in nature and tends to be directed towards the exterior and upwards), *Han Fang Ji* also tends then to treat edema in the upper half of the body and of the wind type.

(d) *Huang Qi Pi* (Cortex Radicis Astragali Membranacei), the outer bark of the Astragalus root, is directed towards the exterior and is more powerful than *Huang Qi* for securing the exterior and stopping perspiration, disinhibiting urination and treating edema.

Han Lian Cao (Herba Ecliptae Prostratae) & *Nu Zhen Zi* (Fructus Ligustri Lucidi)

Individual properties:	
Han Lian Cao	*Nu Zhen Zi*
Nourishes the liver and supplements the kidneys Cools the blood and stops bleeding Enriches yin and blackens the hair Nourishes the lower & upper parts Is harvested during the summer solstice Usual dosage: 6-10g	Nourishes the liver and supplements the kidneys Clears vacuity heat Nourishes liver yin and brightens the eyes Fills the essence and blackens the hair Is harvested during the winter solstice Usual dosage: 6-10g

Properties when combined:

When these two medicinals are combined together, they reinforce one another. Together, they effectively supplement the liver and kidneys, cool the blood and stop bleeding, and blacken the hair.

Major indications of the combination:

1. Liver-kidney vacuity with vacuity heat (1)
2. Vertigo, dizziness, tinnitus, insomnia, and loss of memory due to liver-kidney vacuity with yin and blood not nourishing the upper part of the body (1)
3. Premature greying of hair and beard due to kidney essence vacuity (1)
4. Nosebleed, bleeding gums, hemoptysis, hematemesis, hematuria, and metrorrhagia due to vacuity heat (in turn due to yin vacuity) which forces the blood to move frenetically outside its pathways (1) (2)

Notes:

(1) For these indications, this combination is used in *Er Zhi Wan* (Two Ultimates [*i.e.,* Solstices] Pills). This formula takes its name from the fact that the two medicinal substances forming it are harvested one during the summer solstice (*Han Lian Cao*) and the other during the winter solstice (*Nu Zhen Zi*). For all of these indications, wine-steamed *Nu Zhen Zi* should be prescribed.

(2) The action of *Han Lian Cao* to cool the blood and stop bleeding is not very strong. The combination of *Han Lian Cao* and *Nu Zhen Zi* should, therefore, be strengthened by other medicinals, such as *Sheng Di* (uncooked Radix Rehmanniae), *Mu Dan Pi* (Cortex Radicis Moutan), *Ce Bai Ye* (Cacumen Biotae Orientalis), and *Qian Cao Gen* (Radix Rubiae Cordifoliae).

Comment:

(a) *Han Lian Cao* and *Nu Zhen Zi* are often combined and, as a whole, are less powerful than *Shu Di* (cooked Radix Rehmanniae) or *Gou Qi Zi* (Fructus Lycii Chinensis) for nourishing the blood, yin, or essence. Nevertheless, they have the advantage of not being slimy or difficult to assimilate and, therefore, of not producing stagnation. For this reason, they are purposefully used in case of simultaneous spleen and yin vacuity.

Hong Hua (Flos Carthami Tinctorii) & *Tao Ren* (Semen Pruni Persicae)

Individual properties:	
Hong Hua	**Tao Ren**
Quickens the blood and opens the channels Dispels stasis and stops pain Moves the blood more strongly compared to *Tao Ren* Promotes blood engenderment Tends to dispel stasis in the upper part of the body and in the channels Usual dosage: 6-10g	Breaks blood (stasis) Moistens dryness and lubricates the intestines Dispels stasis more strongly compared to *Hong Hua* Nourishes the blood very slightly Tends to dispel stasis in the lower part of the body, in the abdomen, and in the organs Usual dosage: 6-10g

Properties when combined:

When these two medicinals are combined together, they complement and reinforce each other. Together, they effectively quicken the blood and dispel stasis, engender the blood and stop pain.

Major indications of the combination:

1. Cardiac and chest pain due to heart blood stasis (1)
2. Amenorrhea, dysmenorrhea, menstrual irregularities, and dark menstrual blood with clots due to blood stasis (2)
3. Fixed, stabbing, and severe pain aggravated by pressure due to blood stasis (3)
4. Traumatic injuries with pain and swelling due to blood stasis (4)

Notes:

(1) For these indications, this combination is advantageously reinforced by combining it with *San Qi* (Radix Pseudoginseng), *Dan Shen* (Radix Salviae Miltiorrhizae), *Xie Bai* (Bulbus Allii), and *Gua Lou Pi* (Pericarpium Trichosanthis Kirlowii).

(2) For these indications, this combination is used in *Tao Hong Si Wu Tang* (Persica & Carthamus Four Materials Decoction).

(3) For these indications, this combination is used in many formulas, for example *Xu Fu Zhu Yu Tang* (Blood Mansion Dispel Stasis Decoction), *Tong Qiao Huo Xue Tang* (Open the Orifices & Quicken the Blood Decoction), *Fu Yuan Huo Xue Tang* (Restore the Origin & Quicken the Blood Decoction), *Shen Tong Zhu Yu Tang* (Body Pain Dispel Stasis Decoction), etc.

(4) For this indication, this combination is included in *Xiao Zhong Zhi Tong Tang* (Disperse Swelling & Stop Pain Decoction).

Comments:

(a) It is noteworthy to mention that, just like *Xing Ren* (Semen Pruni Armeniacae), *Tao Ren* is slightly toxic. This toxicity is localized in the superficial skin and the tip of the seed. The preparation, scalded *Tao Ren*, eliminates this toxicity. However, in this form, *Tao Ren* is less powerful for quickening the blood and dispelling stasis.

(b) *Hong Hua*'s action changes depending on its dosage. At a weak dosage of 1-2g per *ji* or prescription, it stimulates the engenderment and transformation of blood. At a moderate dose of 3-5g per *ji*, it harmonizes the blood. At its usual dosage of 6-10g per *ji*, it quickens the blood. At a high dosage of 10-15g per *ji*, it breaks the blood. Thus, the higher the dose, the more powerful it becomes for quickening the blood and dispelling stasis, going from harmonizing to quickening to breaking the blood.

Huang Bai (Cortex Phellodendri) & Ze Xie (Rhizoma Alismatis)

Individual properties:	
Huang Bai	*Ze Xie*
Clears heat and dries dampness Drains fire and resolves toxins Clears vacuity heat Drains fire from the lower burner Clears heat from the yin division Usual dosage: 3-10g	Disinhibits urination and percolates dampness Drains fire from the liver, kidney, and bladder channels Clears damp heat from the lower burner Clears heat from the qi division Usual dosage: 3-10g

Properties when combined:

One dries dampness, while the other percolates dampness.
One drains fire from the lower burner; the other drains dampness from the lower burner.
When these two medicinals are combined together, they clear and drain fire due to yin vacuity. Together, they also clear and eliminate dampness and heat.

Major indications of the combination:

1. Steaming bones, night sweats, and seminal emission due to vacuity fire (1)

2. Inhibited urination and pricking, painful urination due to damp heat in the lower burner (2)

Notes:

(1) For these indications, this combination is present in *Zhi Bai Di Huang Wan* (Anemarrhena & Phellodendron Rehmannia Pills). For these indications, salt mix-fried *Huang Bai* and salt mix-fried *Ze Xie* should be prescribed.

(2) For these indications, salt mix-fried *Huang Bai* and uncooked or salt mix-fried *Ze Xie* should be prescribed.

Huang Bai (Cortex Phellodendri) & Zhi Mu (Rhizoma Anemarrhenae)

Individual properties:	
Huang Bai	*Zhi Mu*
Bitter, cold Consolidates yin (1) Clears heat and dries dampness Drains fire and resolves toxins Clears vacuity heat Tends to eliminate dampness from the lower burner Usual dosage: 6-10g	Sweet, bitter, cold Supplements the kidneys, moistens dryness, enriches yin Clears heat and drains fire Clears the qi division Tends to drain vacuity fire from the lower burner Usual dosage: 6-10g

Properties when combined:

When these two medicinals are combined together, they reinforce and complement each other. Together, they clear heat and enrich yin, drain vacuity fire, resolve toxins, and eliminate dampness in the lower burner.

Major indications of the combination:

1. Evening fever, steaming bones, and night sweats caused by yin vacuity (2)
2. Seminal emission, premature ejaculation, easy erection (in men), and women's excessive thinking about sexual desire due to vacuity fire and hyperactive ministerial fire (2) (3)
3. Dysuria due to yin vacuity and to yang losing its ability to transform (at the level of the bladder) (4)

Notes:

(1) Consolidation of yin is a therapeutic method aimed at clearing and downbearing vacuity fire and thus consolidating the kidney essence in order to treat seminal emission and premature ejaculation caused by kidney yin vacuity and hyperactive ministerial fire.

(2) For these indications, this combination is used in *Zhi Bai Di Huang Wan* (Anemarrhena & Phellodendron Rehmannia Pills).

(3) Ministerial fire is another name for physiological fire which has its source in the life gate but which manifests in the liver, gallbladder, and three burners. It is connected with imperial fire which is the physiological fire of the heart. Ministerial fire warms and nourishes the viscera and bowels in order to ensure their functional activities. However, ministerial fire can flare up out of control, in which case it becomes pathological. In case of liver-kidney yin vacuity, vacuity heat is generated. This may stir up ministerial fire which then becomes hyperactive. This will disturb the kidneys, particularly *vis a vis* their function of storing the essence, thus giving rise to such complaints as seminal emission and premature ejaculation. On the other hand, since sexual desire is a function of ministerial or life gate fire, stirring or hyperactivity of ministerial fire may also give rise to erotic dreams, sexual hyperexcitability, nymphomania, etc.

(4) For this indication, this combination is present in *Zi Shen Wan* (Enrich the Kidneys Pills).

Comment:

(a) For these indications, salt mix-fried *Zhi Mu* and salt mix-fried *Huang Bai* should be prescribed. Salt guides the action of medicinal ingredients towards the lower burner and the kidneys.

Huang Lian (Rhizoma Coptidis Chinensis) & Huang Qin (Radix Scutellariae Baicalensis)

Individual properties:	
Huang Lian	**Huang Qin**
Clears heat and dries dampness	Clears heat and dries dampness
Drains fire and resolves toxins	Drains fire and resolves toxins
Drains heart, stomach & liver fire	Drains lung & large intestine fire
Clears heat and stops bleeding	Clears heat and quiets the fetus
Mainly clears the middle burner but also the upper & lower burners	Clears heat and stops bleeding
Clears heat generated by dampness	Mainly clears the upper burner but also the middle & lower burners
Usual dosage: 3-6g	Eliminates dampness generated by heat
	Usual dosage: 6-10g

Properties when combined:

When these two medicinals are combined together, they effectively clear heat and dry dampness, drain fire and resolve toxins from the upper, middle, and lower burners.

Major indications of the combination:

1. Red, swollen, painful eyes, toothache with red, swollen gums, oral ulcers, and glossitis due to replete heat in the upper and middle burners (1)
2. Vexation and agitation in warm disease with replete heat or due to a breakdown in communication between the heart and kidneys (2)
3. Diarrhea and dysentery due to damp heat (3)
4. Hematemesis and epistaxis due to heat in the blood (1)

Notes:

(1) For these indications, this combination is included in *Xie Xin Tang* (Drain the Heart Decoction). For these indications, wine mix-fried *Huang Lian* and wine mix-fried *Huang Qin* should be prescribed. The alcohol directs the action of these two medicinals towards the upper burner.

(2) For these indications, this combination is used in *Huang Lian Jie Du Tang* (Coptis Resolve Toxins Decoction) and *Huang Lian E Jiao Tang* (Coptis & Donkey Skin Glue Decoction).

(3) For these indications, this combination is used in *Shao Yao Tang* (Peony Decoction).

Comment:

(a) There are two types of *Huang Qin. Ku Qin* (withered Scutellaria) has a light, hollow body. Its color is dark. Its property is floating. Its tropism is to the hand *tai yin* channel. It drains lung fire, clears the upper burner, and drains heat from the muscles and from the exterior. This function is used in the prescription *Jiu Wei Qiang Huo Tang* (Nine Flavors Notopterygium Decoction). *Zi Qin* (young Scutellaria) or *Tiao Qin* (Scutellaria sticks) has a dense, full, hard body. Its color is yellow and slightly green. Its property is sinking. Its tropism is to the hand *yang ming* channel. It drains large intestine fire, clears the lower burner, and treats heat type dysentery. This function is used, for example, in the prescription, *Huang Qin Tang* (Scutellaria Decoction).

Huang Lian (Rhizoma Coptidis Chinensis) & *Mu Xiang* (Radix Auklandiae Lappae)

Individual properties:	
Huang Lian	*Mu Xiang*
Clears heat and dries dampness Drains fire and resolves toxins Clears the liver, stomach & heart Bitter: thickens the intestines and stops diarrhea Cold: cools the blood, resolves toxins, and treats diarrhea or bloody and purulent dysentery Usual dosage: 3-10g	Arouses the spleen and disperses food stagnation Moves the qi, disperses distention, and stops pain Bitter and aromatic: dries dampness Acrid: disperses qi stagnation in the stomach and intestines and treats diarrhea with abdominal pain and tenesmus Usual dosage: 6-10g

Properties when combined:

One is cold and drains; the other is warm and disperses.
When these two medicinals are combined together, they effectively rectify the qi, drain heat, dry dampness, and treat dysentery.

Major indications of the combination:

1. Diarrhea, bloody and purulent dysentery, abdominal pain, and tenesmus due to damp heat and qi stagnation in the large intestine (1)

Note:

(1) For these indications, this combination is used in *Xiang Lian Wan* (Auklandia & Coptis Pills). For these indications, uncooked *Huang Lian* and roasted *Mu Xiang* should be prescribed.

Comment:

(a) For precautions in the use of *Huang Lian*, see comment (a) of the pair *E Jiao* and *Huang Lian* above.

Huang Lian (Rhizoma Coptidis Chinensis) & *Rou Gui* (Cortex Cinnamomi Cassiae)

Individual properties:	
Huang Lian	*Rou Gui*
Bitter, cold Clears heat and dries dampness Drains fire and resolves toxins Clears heat in the heart Drains heart fire Usual dosage: 3-6g	Acrid, hot Warms the middle burner and scatters cold Supplements kidney yang & life gate fire Returns fire to its source (1) Usual dosage: 3-6g

Properties when combined:

One is cold; the other is hot.

One is yin; the other is yang.
One is for the upper burner and the heart; the other is for the middle burner and the kidneys.

When these two medicinals are combined together, they harmonize yin and yang, drain the south (*i.e.*, heart fire) and supplement the north (*i.e.*, kidney yang), and re-establish the interaction between the heart and kidneys.

Major indications of the combination:

1. Insomnia, vexation and agitation due to heart and kidneys not interacting (2)
2. Glossitis, oral ulcers, heart palpitations together with fear of cold, long, clear urination, impotence, and seminal emission due to simultaneous heart fire and kidney yang vacuity

Notes:

(1) If yin becomes vacuous, yin may not control yang anymore. It then tends to float upward. *Rou Gui's* function is to bring back this floating yang to its source or, in other words, towards the lower burner. Of course, in this case, *Rou Gui* must be combined with a substance which nourishes yin in order to re-establish the balance between yin and yang.

(2) The heart corresponds with fire and stores the spirit. The kidneys correspond with water and store the essence. Imperial fire, which is the physiological fire of the heart, descends to warm (*i.e.*, support) kidney yang or true yang. Kidney water, which is true yin, rises to nourish (*i.e.*, support) heart yin. This mutual assistance is the origin of the balance between yin and yang and of the harmonious functioning between south and north, water and fire within the organism. When the interaction between the heart and kidneys is broken, yin and yang, heart and kidneys, spirit and essence are disturbed. This may manifest in many imbalances among which are: 1) Kidney water insufficiency which cannot adequately nourish heart yin and control heart fire which, therefore, blazes. This is the indication for the combination of *Huang Lian* and *E Jiao* which is found in the prescription, *Huang Lian E Jiao Tang* (Coptis & Donkey Skin Glue Decoction). 2) Kidney yang insufficiency which cannot move and upbear kidney water. This then becomes like the water in a swamp, dead and stagnant. In that case, kidney water does not nourish heart yin and

does not control heart fire which rises upward. This is the indication for the combination of *Huang Lian* and *Rou Gui* which can be found in *Jiao Tai Wan* (Peaceful Meeting Pills).

Comments:

(a) Real *Rou Gui* is an expensive medicinal. For reasons unknown to the author, many importers of Chinese medicinal substances sell the culinary quality of Cinnamon, *Gui Pi*. Although this spice is delicious, it has little medicinal value. Its dietary action focuses on the middle burner. In no case does *Gui Pi* reinforce kidney yang or life gate fire. *Guan Gui* (Cortex Tubiformis Cinnamomi Cassiae) is the fine bark of the tree that has lived six to seven years. *Guan Gui* has less oil and its nature is drying. Consequently, it is weaker than *Rou Gui* for supplementing the original qi but is better for warming the middle and drying dampness. *Rou Gui* is for the lower burner and kidneys. *Guan Gui* is for the middle burner and spleen. *Rou Gui Xin* (the heart of *Rou Gui*), also called *Gui Xin*, is Cinnamon bark which has been cleaned of its fine, superficial layer (which is brown and which sometimes looks like cork). *Rou Gui Xin* is believed to be superior for reinforcing heart yang and for re-establishing the interaction between the heart and kidneys. *Rou Gui Mo* or *Rou Gui Mian*, powdered *Rou Gui*, has the advantage of being just as powerful as the whole bark and may be used at a dose of 1-2 g/day. This reduces the cost of the treatment since *Rou Gui* is relatively expensive. This powder can be added five minutes before the end of the decoction or can even be mixed to the decocted liquid just before drinking it.

(b) *Rou Gui* is one of the ingredients in *Shi Quan Da Bu Tang* (Ten [Ingredients] Completely & Greatly Supplementing Decoction). However, contrary to what is often said, in this formula, *Rou Gui* is not used to invigorate yang but to promote the production of qi and blood. *Rou Gui's* action is to warm and reinforce the functions of transformation (mainly at the level of the middle burner and bladder) and thus promote the production of qi and blood. In fact, *Rou Gui* supplements the source qi which takes part in all transformations within the organism and especially in those ruled by the middle burner to engender the qi, blood, and essence. *Shi Quan Da Bu Wan* is the same as *Ba Zhen Tang* (Eight Pearls Decoction) which is the basic formula for supplementing the qi and blood to which have been added *Huang Qi* (Radix Astragali Membranacei) and *Rou Gui*. These additions are to accentuate even more the supplementation of qi and blood. It should also be noted that *Ba Zhen Tang* equals the combination of *Si Wu Tang* (Four Materials Decoction), Chinese medicine's basic formula for supplementing the blood, plus *Si Jun Zi Tang* (Four Gentlemen Decoction), Chinese medicine's basic formula for supplementing the qi.

Huang Lian (Rhizoma Coptidis Chinensis) & *Wu Zhu Yu* (Fructus Evodiae Rutecarpae)

Individual properties:	
Huang Lian	*Wu Zhu Yu*
Clears heat and dries dampness Drains fire and resolves toxins Clears heat and eliminates vexation As the ruler: Clears stomach heat Treats vomiting and acid regurgitation due to liver-stomach disharmony. Drains fire from the liver channel Bitter & cold: drains fire Usual dosage: 3-10g (1)	Warms the middle burner and scatters cold Downbears counterflow and stops vomiting Drains the liver and stops pain As the messenger: Guides the action of *Huang Lian* towards the liver Reinforces the action of *Huang Lian* to treat vomiting and acid regurgitation Drains fire from the liver channel Acrid and hot: opens and frees the flow Usual dosage: 2-5g (1)

Properties when combined:

One is cold, while the other is hot.
One drains, while the other opens.
When these two medicinals are combined together, they effectively drain liver fire, harmonize the stomach, downbear counterflow, and stop pain, acid regurgitation, and vomiting.

Major indications of the combination:

1. Lateral costal pain and distention, nausea, vomiting, acid regurgitation, belching, clamoring stomach, and a bitter taste in the mouth due to liver depression transforming into fire which disturbs the stomach (2)
2. Diarrhea and dysentery due to damp heat

Notes:

(1) Traditionally, this combination is used to treat liver fire causing a liver-stomach disharmony which, in turn, leads to nausea, vomiting, and acid regurgitation. In this case, *Huang Lian* should be prescribed in the larger quantity and *Wu Zhu Yu* in a lesser quantity. However, this pair can also be used in patterns where cold and heat are mixed. In this case, if heat is predominant, the quantity of *Huang Lian* should be proportionally more. If there is concomitant stomach yin vacuity, it is advisable to add *Shi Hu* (Herba Dendrobii). If cold is predominant, the quantity of *Wu Zhu Yu* should be proportionally more. If there is concomitant stomach qi vacuity, it is advisable to add *Dang Shen* (Radix Codonopsitis Pilosulae). If cold and heat are present in identical proportions, the quantities of both medicinals should be equal.

(2) For these indications, this combination is used in *Zuo Jin Wan* (Left Metal Pills).

Huang Lian (Rhizoma Coptidis Chinensis) & Zi Su (Folium Et Caulis Perillae Frutescentis)

Individual properties:	
Huang Lian	**Zi Su**
Bitter, cold, drying, clearing	Acrid, warm, moving, downbearing
Clears heat and dries dampness	Dispels wind cold
Drains fire and resolves toxins	Moves the qi and stops vomiting
Drains stomach, heart & liver fire	Resolves the toxicity of fish & crab
Usual dosage: 3-10g	Usual dosage: 3-10g

Properties when combined:

One is bitter and cold; the other is acrid and warm.
One clears and dries; the other moves and downbears.
When these two medicinals are combined together, they clear stomach heat and, dry dampness, rectify the qi and stop vomiting.

Major indications of the combination:

1. Vomiting and nausea due to stomach heat or damp heat in the middle burner along with qi stagnation in the middle burner (1)
2. Vomiting during pregnancy due to heat or damp heat along with qi stagnation in the middle burner (1)

Note:

(1) For these indications, ginger mix-fried *Huang Lian* should be prescribed.

Comments:

(a) *Zi Su* is the leaf and stem of Perilla. *Zi Su Ye* is the leaf of Perilla. *Zi Su Geng* is the stem of Perilla. *Zi Su Zi* is the seed of Perilla. *Zi Su* resolves the exterior, scatters cold, moves the qi, opens the center, resolves the toxicity from fish and crab, and treats vomiting due to a disharmony of stomach qi and colds due to wind cold. *Zi Su Ye* dispels wind cold more strongly, rectifies the qi, harmonizes the stomach, and particularly treats vomiting occurring in a wind cold pattern and colds and influenza due to wind cold. *Zi Su Geng* moves the qi, opens the center, rectifies the qi, quiets the fetus, and particularly treats vomiting due to pregnancy, threatened miscarriage, and epigastric or abdominal distention. *Zi Su Zi* downbears qi, transforms phlegm, stops cough, and calms asthma.

(b) *Zi Su Ye* and *Zi Su Geng* are incompatible with carp.

(c) *Zi Su Ye* and *Zi Su Geng* are often combined and added to other formulas to treat the plum pit qi or wind cold attacks with food stagnation or vomiting.

Huang Qi (Radix Astragali Membranacei) & *Mu Li* (Concha Ostreae)

Individual properties:	
Huang Qi	*Mu Li*
Sweet, warm, supplementing, upbearing Supplements the qi and upbears yang Secures the exterior and stops perspiration Disinhibits urination and disperses swelling Stops perspiration by supplementing the exterior and filling the pores of the skin Usual dosage: 10-30g	Salty, neutral, astringent, descending Quiets the spirit by its heavy nature Astringent, holds what is escaping Calms the liver and subdues yang Stops perspiration by constraining yin and subduing yang Usual dosage: 15-30g

Properties when combined:

One is a supplement; the other is an astringent. One supplements the qi; the other constrains yin. When these two medicinals are combined together, they effectively supplement the qi and constrain yin, secure the exterior and stop perspiration.

Major indications of the combination:

1. Spontaneous perspiration due to qi or yang vacuity (1)
2. Night sweats due to yin vacuity (2)
3. Spontaneous and nighttime perspiration due to qi and yin vacuity (1)

Notes:

(1) For these indications, this combination is used in *Mu Li San* (Oyster Shell Powder). See also the pairs *Huang Qi* and *Fu Xiao Mai* and *Fu Xiao Mai* and *Ma Huang Gen* above. For these indications, uncooked *Huang Qi* and calcined *Mu Li* should be prescribed. *Mu Li San* (Concha Ostreae Powder) can be prescribed either for spontaneous sweating (which belongs to yang) and also for night sweats (which belongs to yin),

since it treats mainly the branch manifestation, *i.e.*, the perspiration itself. Of the four medicinals within *Mu Li San*, four stop sweating, and three of these are astringent (*Mu Li, Fu Xiao Mai,* and *Ma Huang Gen*). Only one of these is a supplement — *Huang Qi*.

(2) This combination is appropriate for a moderate yin vacuity. In case of vacuity fire, this pair, as well as *Mu Li San*, cannot be used by itself.

Comments:

(a) In comparison, the combination of *Huang Qi* and *Mu Li* appearing in *Mu Li San* is more powerful to stop perspiration and mainly treats the branch manifestation, while the combination of *Huang Qi* and *Bai Zhu* which is contained in *Yu Ping Feng San* (Jade Windscreen Powder) stops perspiration more moderately. However, it is more powerful for supplementing the spleen and exterior qi and mainly treats the root cause.

(b) *Huang Qi Pi* (Cortex Radicis Astragali Membranacei), the outer skin of the Astragalus root, is known to have a marked tropism for the exterior and to be potent for securing the exterior and stopping perspiration.

Huo Xiang (Herba Agastachis Seu Pogostemi) & Pei Lan (Herba Eupatorii Fortunei)

Individual properties:	
Huo Xiang	*Pei Lan*
Acrid, aromatic Strongly clears summerheat (mainly summerheat dampness) Resolves the exterior Transforms dampness and moves the qi Harmonizes the stomach and arouses the spleen Usual dosage: 6-10g	Acrid, aromatic Eliminates summerheat (summerheat dampness and damp heat patterns of warm disease) Transforms dampness & turbidity Opens the stomach and arouses the spleen Goes to the head Usual dosage: 6-10g

Properties when combined:

When these two medicinals are combined together, they effectively transform dampness and turbidity by their aromatic nature, harmonize the middle burner, stop vomiting, eliminate summerheat (and dampness), and stop diarrhea.

Major indications of the combination:

1. Vertigo, head distention, fever with or without perspiration, chest oppression, epigastric distention, nausea, vomiting, abdominal pain, and diarrhea due to external attack of summerheat dampness
2. Spleen pure heat (1)

Note:

(1) Spleen pure heat refers to a rising upward of turbid qi towards the mouth due to spleen heat generated by an excess of fatty and sweet foods. It is accompanied by a sticky, thick feeling in the mouth, a sugary taste in the mouth, abundant salivation, thick, slimy tongue fur, and a slippery pulse.

Comments:

(a) This combination is very effective for its treatment of bad breath or a thick, sticky feeling in the mouth with a sugary taste due to turbid dampness accumulation or turbid dampness transforming into heat.

(b) *Huo Xiang* and *Pei Lan* drain the exterior and eliminate summerheat, transform turbid dampness and stop vomiting. *Huo Xiang* is more powerful for resolving the exterior and eliminating summerheat as well as for stopping vomiting. *Pei Lan* is more powerful for transforming turbid dampness. In addition, *Pei Lan* clears turbid dampness which has transformed into heat and treats spleen pure heat.

(c) *Huo Xiang* is the stem and leaves. *Huo Xiang Ye* (Folium Agastachis Seu Pogostemi) is the leaf. *Huo Xiang Geng* (Caulis Agastachis Seu Pogostemi) is the stem. *Huo Xiang Ye* is more powerful for draining the exterior. *Huo Xiang Geng* is more powerful for harmonizing the stomach and stopping vomiting.

Ji Nei Jin (Endothelium Corneum Gigeriae Galli) & Mang Xiao (Mirabilitum)

Individual properties:	
Ji Nei Jin	**Mang Xiao**
Fortifies the spleen & stomach Disperses food stagnation Secures the essence and reduces urination Transforms stones Usual dosage: 6-10g	Moistens dryness and softens the hard Drains fire and disperses swelling Precipitates downward and frees the flow of the stools Softens & transforms stones Usual dosage: 3-10g

Properties when combined:

When these two medicinals are combined together, they strongly and effectively soften the hard and disperse accumulation, clear heat and transform stones.

Major indications of the combination:

1. Renal lithiasis, urethral lithiasis, and bladder lithiasis (1)

Note:

(1) Clinical experience demonstrates that both substances should not be cooked. In order to fully benefit from their efficacy, they should be reduced to fine powder and mixed. The usual dosage is then 6g of the mixture, twice per day, dissolved in a glass of hot water. For these indications, uncooked *Ji Nei Jin* and uncooked *Mang Xiao* should be prescribed.

Comment:

(a) *Ji Nei Jin* is also effective for biliary lithiasis.

Jie Geng (Radix Platycodi Grandiflori) & Xing Ren (Semen Pruni Armeniacae)

Individual properties:	
Jie Geng	**Xing Ren**
Acrid, diffusing Diffuses the lung qi (1) Disperses phlegm (2) Disinhibits the throat Guides other medicinals towards the lungs Usual dosage: 6-10g	Bitter, draining Downbears lung qi (1) Transforms phlegm (2) Calms asthma and stops cough Moistens the intestines and frees the flow of the stools Usual dosage: 6-10g

Properties when combined:

One upbears; the other downbears.
One diffuses; the other drains.
When these two medicinals are combined

together, they effectively regulate the lungs' function of diffusion and downbearing, transform and disperse phlegm, stop cough and calm asthma.

Major indications of the combination:

1. Cough and/or asthma with chest oppression, profuse phlegm, sore throat, and aphonia due to an attack of external wind (wind cold or wind heat) that disturbs the diffusion and downbearing function of the lungs (3)

Notes:

(1) In fact, *Jie Geng* and *Xing Ren* both have the function of diffusing and downbearing the lung qi. However, *Jie Geng* mainly diffuses, while *Xing Ren* mainly downbears.

(2) In fact, *Jie Geng* and *Xing Ren* both transform and disperse phlegm. However, *Xing Ren* mainly

transforms phlegm, while *Jie Geng* mainly disperses phlegm. Dispersion of phlegm means the promotion of its expectoration.

(3) For these indications, uncooked *Jie Geng* and uncooked *Xing Ren* should be prescribed.

Comments:

(a) *Vis à vis* the toxicity of *Xing Ren*, see comment (d) from the pair *Chuan Bei Mu* and *Xing Ren* above.

(b) For the differences between bitter and sweet *Xing Ren,* see comment (c) from the pair *Chuan Bei Mu* and *Xing Ren* above.

Jie Geng (Radix Platycodi Grandiflori) & *Zhi Ke* (Fructus Citri Aurantii)

Individual properties:	
Jie Geng	**Zhi Ke**
Diffuses the lungs and loosens the diaphragm	Loosens the chest & diaphragm
Disperses phlegm	Rectifies the qi and moves phlegm
Disinhibits the throat and stops cough	Moves the qi and disperses distention
Mainly upbears, but also downbears	Mainly downbears, but also upbears
Mainly regulates the upper burner	Mainly regulates the middle burner but also the
Guides other medicinals towards the lungs	upper burner
Usual dosage: 3-10g	Usual dosage: 3-10g

Properties when combined:

One upbears; the other downbears.
When these two medicinals are combined together, they effectively regulate upbearing and downbearing, regulate the upper and middle burners, diffuse the lung qi, and loosen the chest and diaphragm.

Major indications of the combination:

1. Chest and diaphragm oppression and distention or chest *bi* due to accumulation of phlegm and qi stagnation (1) (2)
2. Epigastric distention, stomach rumbling, and difficult defecation due to disturbance of upbearing and downbearing (2) (3)

Notes:

(1) For these indications, this combination is present in *Jie Geng Zhi Ke Tang* (Platycodon & Aurantium Decoction).

(2) For these indications, one should prescribe uncooked *Jie Geng* and uncooked *Zhi Ke*.

(3) *Zhi Ke* and *Jie Geng* do not moisten the intestines (as does *Huo Ma Ren* [Semen Cannabis Sativae]), do not soften the bowels (as does *Mang Xiao* [Mirabilitum]), and do not precipitate the bowels (as does *Da Huang* [Radix Et Rhizoma Rhei]). However, *Zhi Ke* moves and downbears the qi in the large intestine in order to improve evacuation of stools, while *Jie Geng* diffuses and

downbears the lung qi. The lungs and large intestine have a mutual interior-exterior relationship. When the lung qi correctly descends, the large intestine qi does the same thing, thus promoting the evacuation of stools. Therefore, although *Zhi Ke* and *Jie Geng* at first glance do not have a direct action on the peristalsis, they can treat constipation due to lung-large intestine qi stagnation. Hence, this pair may be used to advantageously reinforce any formula that specifically treats constipation.

Comments:

(a) *Zhi Ke* treats phlegm by moving the qi. If qi circulates fluidly, phlegm is expelled. *Zhi Ke* is well known for downbearing the qi. However, it also upbears the qi and treats, for example, uterine or rectal prolapse.

(b) This combination is remarkably effective for loosening the chest. Therefore, it can be used for any type of affection causing obstruction and blockage of the lung qi and where there is chest pain or chest oppression. This includes patterns such as wind cold, wind heat, summerheat, damp heat, cold dampness, qi stagnation, or accumulation of phlegm. In this case, these two medicinals should be combined with other appropriate medicinals based on the pattern.

(c) *Jie Geng* is incompatible with pork.

Jin Yin Hua (Flos Lonicerae Japonicae) & *Lian Qiao* (Fructus Forsythiae Suspensae)

Individual properties:	
Jin Yin Hua	*Lian Qiao*
Sweet, cold, light, fragrant Clears heat & wind heat Resolves toxins from the blood division Cools the blood and stops dysentery Eliminates heat from the upper part of the body Usual dosage: 10-15g	Bitter, cool, light, floating Clears the heart and upper burner fire Scatters nodulation and disperses swelling Treats skin inflammations Eliminates heat from the whole body Usual dosage: 10-15g

Properties when combined:

Both these medicinals are light, clearing, floating, diffusing, and dissipating. When they are combined together, they strongly and effectively clear heat and resolve toxins.

Major indications of the combination:

1. Colds and influenza due to wind heat (1) (2)
2. Warm diseases with internal heat (1) (2)
3. Headache, eye pain, toothache, sinusitis, and painful, swollen throat due to wind heat (2)
4. Skin eruptions with pruritus due to wind heat (2)
5. Skin inflammation due to heat toxins (2)

Notes:

(1) For these indications, this combination is used in *Yin Qiao San* (Lonicera & Forsythia Powder). However, neither medicinal is acrid or dispels wind heat. By themselves, they cannot expel external wind. They only reinforce other medicinals which have this function. On the other hand, they are often included in formulas for dispelling wind heat in order to prevent the production of heat toxins or to prevent heat from entering deeper into the interior. *Jin Yin Hua* and *Lian Qiao* are able to limit the worsening of colds, influenza, and other illnesses due to wind heat.

(2) For all of these indications, uncooked *Jin Yin Hua* and uncooked *Lian Qiao* should be prescribed.

Comments:

(a) For warm diseases and mild wind heat, the dosage of *Jin Yin Hua* may go to 10-15g per day. But, for severe heat toxins, dysentery, or pyogenic skin infections, 30-60g per day should be prescribed. The more severe is the illness, the higher the dosage can be. *Jin Yin Hua* is one of the few medicinal substances that clears replete heat effectively without having major side effects even at higher dosages. On the other hand, *Lian Qiao's* dosage should not exceed 15g per day, since it may damage stomach yang. Sometimes, in case of severe heat toxins, it can be prescribed up to 30g per day, but for a short period of time and only if the patient does not suffer from a stomach vacuity.

(b) *Lian Qiao* is superior to *Jin Yin Hua* for clearing heat toxins but is not effective for

reinforcing the expelling action of other medicinals which dispel wind heat.

(c) *Lian Qiao Xin* (the heart of *Lian Qiao*) is the small seed contained in the shell of *Lian Qiao*. *Lian Qiao Xin* clears heat toxins which have entered the pericardium causing vexation and agitation, irritability, insomnia, high fever with delirium, mental confusion, and loss of consciousness.

(d) There are two types of *Lian Qiao*. *Qing Lian Qiao* (green *Lian Qiao*) is the fruit which has not completely matured. It is superior for clearing heat, resolving toxins, and treating warm diseases, fever, and erysipelas.

Huang Lian Qiao (yellow *Lian Qiao*) is the mature fruit. It is superior for dispersing abscesses and swelling, scattering nodulation, and treating goitre, subcutaneous nodules, skin inflammations, and carbuncles.

Jin Ying Zi (Fructus Rosae Laevigatae) & *Qian Shi* (Semen Euryalis Ferocis)

Individual properties:	
Jin Ying Zi	**Qian Shi**
Sour, astringent, holds what is escaping Reduces urination Secures the essence Stops diarrhea and abnormal vaginal discharge Usual dosage: 6-12g	Fortifies the spleen and stops diarrhea and abnormal vaginal discharge Supplements the kidneys, secures the essence, and reduces urination Usual dosage: 10-15g

Properties when combined:

One is more astringent; the other is more supplementing.
When these two medicinals are combined together, they effectively supplement the kidneys, secure the essence, and reduce urination, fortify the spleen and stop diarrhea and abnormal vaginal discharge.

Major indications of the combination:

1. Chronic diarrhea due to spleen-kidney vacuity (1) (2)

2. Urinary incontinence, enuresis, frequent micturition, and nocturia due to kidney qi vacuity (1) (3)
3. Chronic white vaginal discharge due to spleen-kidney vacuity (1) (3)
4. Seminal emission and premature ejaculation due to kidney qi not securing (1) (3)

Notes:

(1) For these indications, this combination is included in *Shui Lu Er Xian Dan* (Water & Earth Two Immortals Elixir). *Qian Shi* grows in water (*shui*) and *Jin Ying Zi* grows in earth (*lu*).

(2) For this indication, bran stir-fried *Qian Shi* should be prescribed.

(3) For these indications, uncooked *Qian Shi* should be prescribed.

Comments:

(a) In terms of *Shui Lu Er Xian Dan, xian* is usually translated as immortal and *dan* as elixir. However, *xian* also means something that is divine, celestial. *Dan* expresses the idea that it is a special medicine, typically a pill whose contents are precious. *Dan* is also the color of red vermilion from the alchemist's furnace. Some pills are traditionally coated on the surface with *Zhu Sha* (Cinnabar, a mineral used by alchemists) which gives them a red color, as for example *Tian Wang Bu Xin Dan* (Heavenly Emperor Supplement the Heart Elixir). Therefore, the expression, *xian dan*, conveys the idea of an effective remedy, an elixir of long life which contains precious and efficient substances.

(b) *Jin Ying Zi* and *Qian Shi* are astringent medicinals. Astringent medicinals treat spontaneous, uncontrollable, and excessive leakage (or discharges) of liquids, substances, or qi that normally should stay within the body or which are discharged under certain conditions and control, such as sperm, sweat, saliva, blood, urine, the stools, vaginal secretions, and qi. Thus there are a number of different pathological conditions possibly requiring the use of astringents: seminal emission, premature ejaculation, spontaneous perspiration, night sweats, drooling, hemorrhage, fecal incontinence, chronic diarrhea, nocturia, enuresis, urinary incontinence, abnormal vaginal discharge, and chronic and repetitive cough. When such pathological discharges and leakages require the use of an astringent, their origin is none other than qi vacuity. In such cases, the function of control and containment of the qi is insufficient to maintain these substances in their place or to release them at the appropriate time. Therefore, astringents as a group have the objective of holding what is leaking due to their astringing and securing

property. They exclusively treat the branch manifestation or, in other words, what is spontaneously leaking out. But they do not treat the root cause of the leakage which is qi vacuity. Any of the above conditions may be initially caused by the presence of some evil qi. However, if they continue long enough, eventually chronic disease will damage the containing and securing function of the qi. It is also possible for such leakages and discharges to begin initially from qi vacuity rather than due to the presence of replete evils.

Thus, some precautions are necessary when these medicinals are required. In case of vacuity, these medicinals should be combined with other medicinals which treat the root cause, *i.e.*, which supplement vacuity. In case of simultaneous vacuity and repletion, these medicinals should be combined with some medicinal substances which supplement vacuity and others which eliminate the evils, *i.e.*, those which drain repletion. In case of repletion, these medicinals are categorically contraindicated, since they would otherwise hold the evils within the interior of the body and, therefore, worsen the imbalance.

In clinical practice, astringents are most often used in combination with both other draining and supplementing medicinals. For instance, for enduring and recalcitrant uterine bleeding due to vacuity that forcing the blood outside its pathways, blood stasis also forcing the blood outside its vessels, and kidney qi not securing, one must use medicinals which supplement the kidneys and enrich yin, medicinals which clear heat and cool the blood, medicinals which quicken the blood but also stop bleeding , and medicinals which astringe and secure all at the same time. If any of these are missing, then the effect will not be seen. Therefore, it is extremely important to differentiate mixed repletion and vacuities from simple repletions. If there is a mixed repletion and vacuity with qi having lost its ability to astringe and secure, then astringents are necessary to effect a cure at the same time as draining whatever evils have been identified in the case.

Ju He (Semen Citri Reticulatae) & Li Zhi He (Fructus Litchi Chinensis)

Individual properties:	
Ju He	**Li Zhi He**
Moves the qi	Moves the qi (& blood)
Scatters nodulation	Scatters cold
Stops pain	Stops pain
Directed towards the *jue yin* channel and the qi division	Directed towards the *jue yin* channel and the blood division
Directed towards the lower burner, into the kidney channel, and treats *shan* (1)	Directed towards the lower burner, the kidney channel, and treats *shan* (1)
Usual dosage: 6-10g	Usual dosage: 6-10g

Properties when combined:

One is directed towards the qi division; the other towards the blood division.

When these two medicinals are combined together, they are directed towards the liver channel and especially to the region of the pelvis. They effectively scatter cold, scatter nodulation, and stop pain.

Major indications of the combination:

1. Inguinal hernia, swelling and pain of the testicles, and scrotal hernia all due to cold qi congealing and stagnating in the liver channel (2)
2. Piercing pain in the pelvis due to qi stagnation and blood stasis (2)
3. Masses in the pelvis (chronic salpingitis, chronic salpingo-ovaritis, chronic adnexititis, ovarian cysts, endometriosis, and fibroids) due to qi stagnation and blood stasis (2)
4. Abnormal vaginal discharge due to vacuity cold (2)

Notes:

(1) The term *shan* is used in a number of different ways. First, it may be a generic term for all diseases of the scrotum and testicles. Secondly, it may refer specifically to hernias and particularly to inguinal hernias. Third, it can also cover severe abdominal pain associated to anuria and constipation. Moreover, the term cold *shan* may indicate either of two pathologies: 1) Severe periumbilical pain and abdominal spasms together with spontaneous cold perspiration, fear of cold, cold limbs, a deep, tight pulse, and sometimes, in severe cases, numbness of the limbs and generalized stiffness due to a stagnation and congelation of cold evils in the interior of the abdomen. 2) Scrotal or testicular disease due to stagnation and congelation of cold dampness in the liver channel with pain, contracture, swelling, and hardening of the testicles, pain radiating toward the scrotum worsened by cold, etc.

(2) For all of these indications, salt mix-fried *Ju He* and salt mix-fried *Li Zhi He* should be prescribed. Salt guides the action of these medicinals toward the lower burner, toward the pelvis, and toward the kidneys. In addition, salt promotes the softening nodulations in the treatment of *shan*.

Comment:

(a) This combination is used with success in strangury patterns, particularly for stone strangury and qi strangury (qi stagnation type), in order to counteract piercingly painful urination and spasms and contractures in the pelvis. For these purposes, this pair is an auxiliary treatment and should be added to other standard formulas that treat strangury.

Ju Hong (Epicarpium Rubrum Citri Reticulatae) & Zi Wan (Radix Asteris Tatarici)

Individual properties:	
Ju Hong	**Zi Wan**
Scatters cold and rectifies the qi Resolves the exterior Dries dampness and transforms phlegm Disperses food stagnation and disperses distention Warm, drying, aromatic: tends to dry dampness and transform phlegm causing cough and moves the qi to disperse phlegm Usual dosage: 3-6g	Moistens the lungs and downbears counterflow Eliminates phlegm and stops cough Drains lung heat Warm but not hot; acrid but not drying; moistening but not cold Tends to disperse qi stagnation in the lungs, moisten the lungs, and disperse phlegm stagnating in the lungs Usual dosage: 6-10g

Properties when combined:

One dries; the other moistens.
One moves the qi; the other downbears the qi.
One transforms phlegm; the other disperses phlegm.
When these two medicinals are combined together, they effectively dry dampness and transform phlegm without drying the lungs, rectify the qi and stop cough.

Major indications of the combination:

1. Cough with profuse phlegm and chest oppression due to accumulation of phlegm and qi stagnating in the lungs (1)
2. Cough with itchy throat, low-grade fever, fear of cold, and profuse phlegm due to wind evils attacking the lungs (2)
3. Cough of internal or external origin due to cold or heat, repletion or vacuity (1)

Notes:

(1) In case of vacuity or dryness of the lungs, honey mix-fried Ju Hong and honey mix-fried Zi Wan should be prescribed.

(2) For these indications, this combination is included in Zhi Sou San (Stop Cough Powder).

Comments:

(a) In case of cough due to accumulation of phlegm in the lungs, once the phlegm is eliminated, the cough automatically calms down. To disperse phlegm, first disperse the phlegm already in place. Zi Wan does this through promoting expectoration, and Ju Hong does this by promoting metabolic transformation. Then, one should prevent the production of new phlegm. That is Ju Hong's role. To transform phlegm, it is necessary to follow three therapeutic strategies: 1) transform, 2) move, 3) fortify. For a fuller discussion of these three, see comment (a) of the pair Ban Xia and Chen Pi.

(b) Ju Hong and Ju Pi (Chen Pi) come from the same peel of the mandarin orange fruit. Ju Pi is the whole peel, while Ju Hong is the external and red-orange part of the peel. The internal part of the peel is white and has been removed. It corresponds to another medicinal substance, Ju Bai. Ju Hong and Ju Pi have analogous actions. However, Ju Hong dries dampness and transforms phlegm more strongly. In addition, it scatters wind and cold.

Ju Hua (Flos Chrysanthemi Morifolii) & *Sang Ye* (Folium Mori Albi)

Individual properties:	
Ju Hua	***Sang Ye***
Clears heat and dispels wind Clears the liver, brightens the eyes, and clears the head Calms the liver and extinguishes wind Directed to the eyes & liver channel Superior for clearing heat & the liver Usual dosage: 6-10g	Dispels wind heat Diffuses the lungs and drains heat from the lungs, moistens the lungs and stops cough Clears the liver and brightens the eyes Directed to the lungs network vessels Superior for dispelling wind Usual dosage: 6-10g

Properties when combined:

One mainly clears heat; the other mainly dispels wind.
One is for the liver; the other is for the lungs.
When these two medicinals are combined together, they effectively dispel wind heat, clear the liver and brighten the eyes, clear the lungs and stop cough.

Major indications of the combination:

1. Fever, slight fear of wind, light perspiration, cough, headache, and slight thirst due to wind heat attacking the lungs (1)
2. Headache, vertigo, photophobia, and red, swollen, painful eyes due to ascendant hyperactivity of liver yang (2)

Notes:

(1) For these indications, this combination is present in *Sang Ju Yin* (Morus & Chrysanthemum Drink). For these indications, uncooked (yellow) *Ju Hua* and uncooked *Sang Ye* should be prescribed.

(2) For these indications, stir-fried till scorched (white) *Ju Hua* and stir-fried till scorched *Sang Ye* should be prescribed.

Comments:

(a) *Bai Ju Hua* (white *Ju Hua*) tends to be sweet and slightly bitter. It is also called *Gan Ju Hua* (sweet *Ju Hua*). *Bai Ju Hua* dispels wind heat moderately, but it calms the liver and brightens the eyes. It is used for eye disorders, vertigo, headache, and tinnitus due to liver-kidney yin vacuity causing liver yang hyperactivity. (See the pair *Gou Qi Zi* and *Ju Hua* above.) *Huang Ju Hua* (yellow *Ju Hua*) tends to be bitter and slightly sweet. It is stronger than *Bai Ju Hua* for dispelling wind heat and it expels wind heat attacking the lungs. It is used for colds, influenza, and cough due to wind heat. Therefore, *Huang Ju Hua* should be prescribed for cases of wind heat, *Bai Ju Hua* should be prescribed for cases of liver yang hyperactivity.

(b) *Sang Ye*, *Sang Zhi* (Ramulus Mori Albi), *Sang Shen Zi* (Fructus Mori Albi), and *Sang Bai Pi* (Cortex Radicis Mori Albi) all come from the same tree, the white mulberry tree (*Morus alba L.*). *Sang Ye*, the leaves of the mulberry tree, dispels wind heat, clears the liver, and brightens the eyes. *Sang Zhi*, the young twigs of the mulberry tree, drain wind dampness, open the network vessels, and disinhibit the joints. *Sang Shen Zi*, the ripe fruits of the mulberry tree, supplement yin and blood, nourish the liver and kidneys, moisten the intestines and free the flow of the stools. *Sang Bai Pi*, the root bark of the mulberry tree, clears the lungs, calms asthma, disinhibits urination, and disperses swelling.

(c) For the dosage of *Ju Hua*, see comment (a) of the pair *Gou Qi Zi* and *Ju Hua*.

Lian Zi (Semen Nelumbinis Nuciferae) & Qian Shi (Semen Euryalis Ferocis)

Individual properties:	
Lian Zi	**Qian Shi**
Sweet, astringent Fortifies the spleen and stops diarrhea Supplements the kidneys and secures the essence Nourishes the heart and quiets the spirit Promotes the interaction between the heart & kidneys Superior for supplementing the spleen and nourishing the heart Usual dosage: 6-12g	Sweet, astringent Supplements the kidneys, secures the essence, and reduces urination Fortifies the spleen and stops diarrhea Eliminates dampness and stops vaginal discharge Superior for supplementing the kidneys and securing the essence Usual dosage: 10-15g

Properties when combined:

When these two medicinals are combined together, they mutually reinforce each other. Together, they effectively fortify the spleen and stop diarrhea, supplement the kidneys and secure the essence, reduce urination and stop abnormal vaginal discharge.

Major indications of the combination:

1. Enduring diarrhea due to spleen vacuity (1)
2. Enduring vaginal discharge due to spleen vacuity causing accumulation of dampness (2)
3. Seminal emission and premature ejaculation due to kidney qi vacuity (3)
4. Frequent urination, incontinence, and enuresis due to kidney qi vacuity (4)

Notes:

(1) For this indication, stir-fried till yellow *Lian Zi* and bran stir-fried *Qian Shi* should be prescribed.

(2) For this indication, stir-fried till yellow *Lian Zi* and uncooked *Qian Shi* should be prescribed.

(3) For these indications, this combination is used in *Jin Suo Gu Jing Wan* (Golden Lock Secure the Essence Pills). For these indications, stir-fried till yellow *Lian Zi* and uncooked *Qian Shi* should be prescribed.

(4) For this indication, stir-fried till yellow *Lian Zi* and uncooked *Qian Shi* should be prescribed.

Comments:

(a) It should be noted that *Lian Zi* and *Qian Shi* are astringent but also supplementing. Therefore, they simultaneously treat the branch manifestations and the root cause. However, their supplementing action is relatively weak and must be reinforced by supplementing medicinals of greater strength.

(b) The lotus (*Nelumbo nucifera*) is a plant which gives an impressive number of medicinal substances. Not less than 10 are known (without mentioning the different preparations which multiply the possibility). *Lian Zi* or *Lian Rou* is the seed of the lotus (Semen Nelumbinis Nuciferae). It fortifies the spleen and stops diarrhea, supplements the kidneys and secures the essence, nourishes the heart and quiets the spirit. *Lian Zi Xin* or *Lian Xin* is the green sprout of the lotus seed (Plumula Nelumbinis Nuciferae). It drains heart fire, eliminates vexation, and quiets the spirit. *Liang Fang* or *Lian Ke* is the receptacle containing the lotus seeds (Receptaculum Nelumbinis Nuciferae). It dispels stasis and stops bleeding. *Lian Xu* is the stamen of the lotus flower (Stamen Nelumbinis Nuciferae). It secures the kidneys, constrains the essence, and stops bleeding by astringing. *Lian Hua* is the bud of the lotus flower (Flos Nelumbinis Nuciferae). It quickens the blood and stops bleeding, eliminates dampness and clears summerheat. *He Ye* is the lotus leaf (Folium Nelumbinis Nuciferae). It clears summerheat and eliminates dampness, upbears clear yang and stops bleeding. *He Ye Di* or *He Di* is the superior part of the leafstalk and the base of the lotus leaf (Pediculus Nelumbinis Nuciferae). It harmonizes the stomach, quiets the fetus, stops bleeding, stops abnormal vaginal discharge, upbears clear yang, and treats diarrhea.

He Geng is the lotus leaf stalk (Petiolus Nelumbinis Nuciferae). It moves the qi and opens the center, loosens the chest and clears summerheat. *Ou Jie* is the knot of the lotus rhizome (Nodus Nelumbinis Nuciferae). It cools the blood and stops bleeding by astringing. *Ou* is the lotus rhizome (Rhizoma Nelumbinis Nuciferae). It clears heat and cools the blood, dispels stasis and stops thirst.

Long Gu (Os Draconis) & *Mu Li* (Concha Ostreae)

Individual properties:	
Long Gu	*Mu Li*
Sweet, astringent, neutral Fossilized bone and, therefore, heavy by nature Calms the liver and subdues yang Quiets the spirit & ethereal soul with its heavy nature Stops tremors Stops perspiration and secures the essence Stops bleeding and stops diarrhea Promotes tissue regeneration and speeds up healing Normal dosage: 15-30g	Salty, astringent, cold A shell and, therefore, heavy by nature Calms the liver and subdues yang Quiets the spirit & corporeal soul with its heavy nature Stops tremors Stops perspiration and secures the essence Stops bleeding and stops diarrhea Softens the hard and scatters nodulations Treats gastric hyperacidity Normal dosage: 15-30g

Properties when combined:

When these two medicinals are combined together, they mutually reinforce each other. Together, they effectively calm the liver and subdue yang, quiet the spirit, soften the hard and scatter nodulation, and hold and constrain (abnormal discharge).

Major indications of the combination:

1. Vexation and agitation, heart palpitations, insomnia, loss of memory, dizziness, vertigo, photophobia, and tinnitus due to liver yang hyperactivity harassing the spirit (1) (2)
2. Arterial high blood pressure due to yin vacuity causing liver yang hyperactivity (2)
3. Continuous diarrhea or dysentery (3)
4. Urinary incontinence, spermatorrhea, metrorrhagia, abnormal vaginal discharge, and excessive perspiration due to vacuity (3)

5. Pain and distention in the lateral costal region (4)

Notes:

(1) The ethereal soul is made out of yang essence, while the corporeal soul is made out of yin essence. *Long Gu* moves towards the liver and quiets the ethereal soul. *Mu Li* moves towards the lungs and strengthens the corporeal soul. If the ethereal and corporeal souls are quiet and strong, the spirit is steady and peaceful. It is amusing to note that one of the secondary meanings of the character *gu* (bone) means *hun* or the ethereal soul according to the *Han Yu Da Zi Dian (The Large Dictionary of the Chinese Language)*, while *Long Gu* (dragon bone) quiets the ethereal soul. Thus the *hun* (*gu*) treats the *hun*!

(2) For these indications, one should prescribe uncooked *Long Gu* and uncooked *Mu Li*.

(3) For these indications, one should prescribe calcined *Long Gu* and calcined *Mu Li*.

(4) The combination of distention and pain in the lateral costal region is essentially caused by liver depression qi stagnation. To treat this condition, it is necessary to prescribe medicinals that move and drain the liver qi. In this case, since *Long Gu* and *Mu Li* have astringent natures and, therefore, have actions opposite to moving the qi, why do they treat this problem? Liver depression qi stagnation often has its origin in emotional upsetment, irritability, mental depression, anger, and frustration. *Long Gu* and *Mu Li* constrain and hold liver fire and subdue liver yang, calm the liver and quiet the spirit. It is by these means that they rectify the liver and prevent liver depression qi stagnation. They do not treat liver depression qi stagnation directly, but they prevent the onset of stagnation and the transformation of liver depression into liver fire or liver yang hyperactivity.

Comments:

(a) *Long Gu* is incompatible with carp.

(b) *Long Gu* and *Mu Li* have similar actions: They quiet the spirit by their heavy nature, calm the liver and subdue yang, and are astringents. However, *Long Gu* is superior for quieting the spirit, stopping tremors, and holding what is escaping. *Mu Li* is superior for calming the liver and subduing yang.

Ma Huang (Herba Ephedrae) & *She Gan* (Rhizoma Belamcandae)

Individual properties:	
Ma Huang	**She Gan**
Acrid, warm, dissipating Scatters cold and resolves the exterior Diffuses the lung qi Calms asthma Disinhibits urination and disperses swelling Usual dosage: 3-6g	Bitter, cold, downbearing Clears heat and resolves toxins Downbears the lung qi Disperses phlegm Disinhibits the throat Usual dosage: 6-10g

Properties when combined:

One is warm; the other is cold.
One diffuses; the other downbears.
When these two medicinals are combined together, they combine the diffusion and downbearing methods. Together, they diffuse the lungs and downbear the qi, disperse phlegm and calm asthma.

Major indications of the combination:

1. Asthma with asthmatic wheezing due to accumulation of phlegm rheum that blocks the circulation of lung qi which then counterflows (1)

Note:

(1) For these indications, this combination is found in *She Gan Ma Huang Tang* (Belamcanda & Ephedra Decoction).

Comments:

(a) For the treatment of asthma, one should prescribe honey mix-fried *Ma Huang*.

(b) *She Gan* is the key medicinal substance for the treatment of throat inflammation due to heat toxins together with accumulation of phlegm in the throat. Together with *Ma Huang*, *She Gan* expels phlegm accumulated in the lungs and throat causing cough or asthma with stertor and asthmatic wheezing.

Ma Huang (Herba Ephedrae) & Shi Gao (Gypsum Fibrosum)

Individual properties:	
Ma Huang	**Shi Gao**
Acrid, warm, floating, diffusing Its stem is hollow; its tendency is to diffuse Diffuses the lung qi and calms asthma Opens the interstices and promotes perspiration Dispels wind cold Warms and transforms the bladder (*i.e.*, urination) Disinhibits urination and disperses swelling Usual dosage: 3-10g	Acrid, cold, downbearing, draining Its body is heavy; its tendency is to downbear Clears heat and drains fire Resolves heat from the muscles Drains lung heat Clears stomach heat Engenders fluids and stops thirst Usual dosage: 15-60g

Properties when combined:

One is warm; the other is cold.
One scatters cold; the other clears heat.
One diffuses; the other downbears.
When these two medicinals are combined together, they complement and mutually reinforce one another. Together, they effectively diffuse the lungs and calm asthma, disinhibit urination and disperse swelling, clear heat and drain fire.

Major indications of the combination:

1. Wind water or edema with fever, fear of wind, edematous face, eyes, and limbs, joint pain, oliguria, and a floating pulse due to external wind (1) (2)
2. Generalized edema with abdominal repletion, dyspnea, and a deep, slow pulse due to spleen-kidney yang vacuity (2)
3. Stone water or stone edema with the pelvis swollen and hard as a stone, pain and distention in the lateral costal region, edema, abdominal distention, and a deep pulse due to accumulation of yin cold in the liver and kidneys (2)
4. Cough, asthma with fast breathing, sometimes fever and perspiration, thirst, a red tongue with yellow fur, and a slippery, rapid pulse due to lung heat (3)

Notes:

(1) For these indications, this combination is used in *Yue Bi Tang* (Maidservant from Yue Decoction). This formula is composed essentially of *Ma Huang*, *Shi Gao*, and *Gan Cao* (Radix Glycyrrhizae). According to the physician, Zhao Lian-yun, honey mix-fried *Ma Huang* is sweet and warm, enters the hand and foot *tai yin* channels, moves the qi of the three yin channels, and moves towards the skin where it drains yin cold. Uncooked *Shi Gao* is sweet and cold, enters the hand and foot *yang ming* channels, moves the qi of the three yang channels, and moves towards the muscles and flesh where it drains wind and heat. Uncooked *Gan Cao* is sweet in flavor, belongs to earth, and, therefore, possesses a harmonizing property. *Gan Cao* harmonizes the warm nature of *Ma Huang* and the cold nature of *Shi Gao*. It harmonizes yin and yang and allows both medicinals of opposite nature to work together.

(2) For these indications, uncooked *Ma Huang* and uncooked *Shi Gao* should be prescribed.

(3) For these indications, this combination is used in *Ma Xing Shi Gan Tang* (Ephedra, Armeniaca, Gypsum & Licorice Decoction). For these indications, honey mix-fried *Ma Huang* and uncooked *Shi Gao* should be prescribed.

Comments:

(a) The sinking nature of *Shi Gao* controls the floating and sudorific nature of *Ma Huang*. As a result, *Ma Huang* more effectively downbears the lung qi and calms the asthma. This is reinforced by the honey mix-frying preparation.

(b) This combination is remarkable for any type of edema, damp accumulation, or asthma associated with an external pattern together with internal heat. When damage to the exterior is light and heat is severe (fever, great thirst, perspiration), one should prescribe a stronger dosage of *Shi Gao*, *i.e.*, six times that of *Ma Huang* (6:1). When damage to the exterior is severe and heat is light (absence of perspiration, light fever, shivering), one should prescribe a lesser dosage of *Shi Gao*, *i.e.*, three times that of *Ma Huang* (3:1).

Ma Huang (Herba Ephedrae) & *Shu Di* (Cooked Radix Rehmanniae)

Individual properties:	
Ma Huang	*Shu Di*
Acrid, warm Sudorific, resolves the exterior Diffuses the lungs and calms asthma Disinhibits urination and disperses swelling Strong dissipating property which tends to damage the correct qi Usual dosage: 3-9g	Sweet, warm Supplements the blood and engenders fluids Nourishes the liver and enriches the kidneys Supplements the kidneys and boosts the essence Nourishing and greasy property which tends to engender dampness and cause stomach qi stagnation Usual dosage: 6-15g

Properties when combined:

One dissipates; the other nourishes.
One dries; the other moistens.
One is for the lungs; the other is for the kidneys. When these two medicinals are combined together, metal and water generate each other. Together, they simultaneously address the branch manifestations and root cause. Together, they supplement the kidneys and boost the essence, diffuse the lungs and calm asthma, and scatter nodulations and disperse lumps.

Major indications of the combination:

1. Chronic asthma with yin (or blood) vacuity (1)
2. Asthma in women during menstruation (1)
3. Chronic asthma with kidney vacuity and phlegm cold (1)
4. Subcutaneous nodules, carbuncles, abscesses, toe gangrene (*tuo ju*: necrosis of the toes due to arterial sclerosis, a sign observed in obstructive arteriosclerosis, thromboangiitis obliterans), and swollen, painful knees of the yin type due to cold and dampness obstructing the channels (2) (3)

Notes:

(1) For these indications, honey mix-fried *Ma Huang* should be prescribed.

(2) For these indications, this combination is used in *Yang He Tang* (Yang Harmonizing Decoction).

(3) The process of this type of imbalance is as follows: Vacuity of qi and blood predisposes one to the penetration of the evil cold. When evil cold lodges in the superficial aspects of the body, yang is damaged causing a yang vacuity. Cold blocks the circulation of qi and blood at the level of the muscles and flesh, sinews and bones, joints and blood vessels. This pathologic process is based on vacuity. Therefore, it is yin by nature (in comparison to other pathological processes based on repletion and, therefore, yang by nature). The treatment plan consists then in draining the evil cold located in the superficial aspects of the body. This is the role of *Ma Huang* (3g/day). In addition, one must nourish the blood and yin. This is the role of *Shu Di* (15g/day). And further, one should also supplement yang, for instance using *Lu Jiao* (Cornu Cervi) or *Rou Gui* (Cortex Cinnamomi Cassiae).

Comments:

(a) The acrid and dissipating characteristics of

Ma Huang alleviate the slimy and obstructing characteristics of *Shu Di* and allow supplementation without causing qi stagnation. Conversely, the nourishing and moistening characteristics of *Shu Di* alleviate the dissipating and drying characteristics of *Ma Huang* and allow for diffusion and draining without damaging the correct qi.

(b) *Shu Di* is incompatible with any type of animal blood, onions, chives, turnips, radishes, and garlic.

Ma Huang (Herba Ephedrae) & *Xing Ren* (Semen Pruni Armeniacae)

Individual properties:	
Ma Huang	**Xing Ren**
Acrid, dissipating Diffuses the lung qi Calms asthma Induces perspiration and resolves the exterior Usual dosage: 3-10g	Bitter, downbearing Downbears the lung qi Stops cough and calms asthma Moistens the intestines and frees the flow of the stools Usual dosage: 3-10g

Properties when combined:

One diffuses; the other downbears.
One opens; the other drains.
When these two medicinals are combined together, they complement and mutually assist each other. Together, they rectify the lungs qi, stop cough, and calm asthma.

Major indications of the combination:

1. Wind cold pattern (1)
2. Cough and asthma due to wind cold (2)
3. Cough and asthma due to lung heat (3)

Notes:

(1) For this pattern, this combination is used in *Ma Huang Tang* (Ephedra Decoction).

(2) For these indications, this combination is used in *San Ao Tang* (Three [Ingredients] Rough & Ready Decoction).

(3) For these indications, *Ma Huang* and *Xing Ren* should be combined with *Shi Gao* (Gypsum Fibrosum) as in *Ma Xing Shi Gan Tang* (Ephedra, Armeniaca, Gypsum & Licorice Decoction).

Comments:

(a) For the differences between bitter *Xing Ren* and sweet *Xing Ren*, see comment (c) of the pair *Chuan Bei Mu* and *Xing Ren* above.

(b) Regarding the toxicity of *Xing Ren*, see comment (d) of the pair *Chuan Bei Mu* and *Xing Ren* above.

(c) Regarding the sudorific action of *Ma Huang Tang* and cautions in its use, see comment (a) from the pair *Gui Zhi* and *Ma Huang* above.

(d) To stop cough and calm asthma, it is advantageous to prescribe honey mix-fried *Ma Huang*.

Mai Men Dong (Tuber Ophiopogonis Japonici) & *Tian Men Dong* (Tuber Aspargi Cochinensis)

Individual properties:	
Mai Men Dong	*Tian Men Dong*
Sweet, slightly cold Clears heat and nourishes yin Moistens the lungs, stops cough, and transforms phlegm Nourishes the stomach and engenders fluids Clears the heart and eliminates vexation Nourishes, moistens & clears the upper & middle burners Usual dosage: 10-15g	Sweet, very cold Clears heat and nourishes yin Moistens the lungs and stops cough Nourishes the kidneys and downbears vacuity fire Moistens the intestines and frees the flow of the stools Nourishes, moistens & clears the upper and lower burners Usual dosage: 10-15g

Properties when combined:

When these two medicinals are combined together, sweet and cold clear and moisten. Together, they nourish yin and moisten dryness, clear vacuity heat (or replete heat damaging yin) of the lungs, stomach, and kidneys.

Major indications of the combination:

1. Dry mouth, thirst, dry cough with little phlegm, fever, and vexation due to vacuity heat (1)
2. Cough with hemoptysis due to heat damaging the network vessels of the lungs (1)
3. Upper thirsting & wasting with excessive drinking, thirst, and dry throat and tongue due to lung heat damaging the fluids
4. Whooping cough damaging lung yin (2)

Notes:

(1) For these indications, this combination is used in *Tian Dong Gao* (Asparagus Syrup) and *Er Dong Gao* (Two *Dong* Syrup).

(2) This combination completes the classical formulas treating hundred day cough, *i.e.*,

whooping cough, when there is damage to lung yin.

Comments:

(a) *Mai Men Dong* and *Tian Men Dong* are incompatible with carp.

(b) These two medicinal substances are very often associated and called in prescriptions, *Er Dong*, the two *Dong*. They are also often referred to as *Tian Mai Dong*, *Tian (Men) Dong* and *Mai (Men) Dong*.

(c) *Mai Men Dong* and *Tian Men Dong* have similar actions. Both nourish yin, clear and moisten the lungs, moisten the intestines and free the flow of the stools, clear and nourish the heart, and quiet the spirit. However, *Mai Men Dong* has a marked tropism for the upper and middle burners. Therefore, it is favorably prescribed for lung and stomach yin vacuity, and it is superior for nourishing the heart and quieting the spirit. *Tian Men Dong* has a marked tropism for the upper and lower burners. It is favorably prescribed for lung-kidney yin vacuity, and it is superior for clearing and moistening.

Mo Yao (Resina Myrrhae) & Ru Xiang (Resina Olibani)

Individual properties:	
Mo Yao	**Ru Xiang**
Neutral, bitter, draining Quickens the blood and breaks stasis Disperses swelling and stops pain Mainly quickens the blood and dispels stasis Usual dosage: 3-10g	Warm, aromatic, acrid, moving Moves the blood and qi, quickens the blood Soothes the sinews and frees the flow of the network vessels Disperses swelling and stops pain Mainly moves the qi and quickens the blood Usual dosage: 3-10g

Properties when combined:

One tends to rectify the blood; the other to rectify the qi.
When these two medicinals are combined together, they complement and mutually reinforce each other. Together, they effectively move the qi and quicken the blood, dispel stasis, free the flow of the viscera and bowels and channels and network vessels, quicken the network vessels, disperse swelling, stop pain, and constrain (weeping) sores and engender muscle (*i.e.*, flesh).

Major indications of the combination:

1. Pain in the epigastrium, abdomen, hypochondria, and /or heart due to qi and blood stasis and stagnation in the viscera and bowels or channels and network vessels
2. Amenorrhea, dysmenorrhea, or postpartum abdominal pain due to blood stasis
3. Rheumatic complaints due to wind dampness causing qi and blood stagnation and stasis in the network vessels
4. Wounds, scars, and skin inflammations with blood stasis and necrotic tissue
5. Traumatic injuries with pain, swelling, and redness due to qi stagnation and blood stasis (1)

Note:

(1) For traumatic injury to the chest, lateral costal region, low back, or abdomen, *Ru Xiang* and *Mo Yao* are favorably combined with *Si Gua Luo* (Fasciculus Vascularis Luffae Cylindricae). For traumatic injury to the limbs (bones, sinews), *Ru Xiang* and *Mo Yao* are favorably combined with

Sang Zhi (Ramulus Mori Albi).

Comments:

(a) Uncooked *Mo Yao* and uncooked *Ru Xiang* are irritating to the stomach's mucous membranes and cause nausea and vomiting. This form of these medicinals should only be used for external application. When used in decoction, these two medicinals are stir-fried or prepared with vinegar.

(b) The usual dosages of these medicinals should be strictly respected, since overdosing with *Mo Yao* and *Ru Xiang* may cause nausea, vomiting, loss of appetite, heartburn, or discomfort in the stomach.

(c) *Ru Xiang* and *Mo Yao* have similar actions. They are very often combined and in prescriptions are often collectively called *Ru Mo*, *i.e.*, *Ru Xiang* and *Mo Yao*.

(d) Li Shi-zhen said , "*Ru Xiang* quickens the blood; *Mo Yao* breaks the blood." Yang Qing-yu said, "If the patient cannot stretch out their joints, *Ru Xiang* should be added to extend the sinews." These two medicinals quicken the blood and stop pain, disperse swelling and promote tissue regeneration. However, *Mo Yao* is superior for quickening the blood, breaking stasis, and stopping pain. *Ru Xiang* is superior for simultaneously moving the qi and blood and freeing the flow of the network vessels to treat *bi* with loss of articular mobility and contracture of the sinews.

Pu Gong Ying (Herba Taraxaci Mongolici Cum Radice) & Zi Hua Di Ding (Herba Violae Yedoensis Cum Radice)

Individual properties:	
Pu Gong Ying	**Zi Hua Di Ding**
Bitter, cold Tropism: the qi division Clears heat and resolves toxins Disperses welling abscesses, softens the hard, and scatters nodulation Usual dosage: 10-30g	Bitter, acrid, cold Tropism: the blood division Clears heat, cools the blood, and resolves toxins Disperses and scatters welling abscesses & swelling Usual dosage: 10-30g

Properties when combined:

When these two medicinals are combined together, they mutually reinforce each other. Together, they effectively clear heat and resolve toxins, disperse and scatter welling abscesses and swelling, and stop pain.

Major indications of the combination:

1. Pyogenic cutaneous inflammations and erysipelas due to heat toxins (1) (2)
2. Mastitis and appendicitis due to heat toxins (1)
3. Urinary tract infection due to heat toxins (1)
4. Pyogenic inflammatory illnesses due to heat toxins (1) (2) (3)

Notes:

(1) In all cases, if the injury is serious, it is necessary to prescribe a higher dosage of each of the two medicinals, i.e., 30-60g per day.

(2) For these indications, this combination is used in Wu Wei Xiao Du Yin (Five Flavors Disperse Toxins Drink).

(3) For lung abscess, this pair is favorably combined with Yu Xing Cao (Herba Houttuyniae Cordatae Cum Radice), Bai Jiang Cao (Herba Patriniae Heterophyllae), and Lu Gen (Rhizoma Phragmitis Communis). For intestinal abscess, i.e., appendicitis, this pair is favorably combined with Bai Jian Cao, Hong Teng (Caulis Sargentodoxae), Da Huang (Radix Et Rhizoma Rhei), and Mu Dan (Cortex Radicis Moutan). For breast welling abscess, i.e., mastitis, this pair is favorably combined with Gua Lou (Fructus Trichosanthis Kirlowii), Lian Qiao (Fructus Forsythiae Suspensae), Wang Bu Liu Xing (Semen Vaccariae Segetalis), and Lou Lu (Radix Rhapontici Seu Echinopsis). For severe inflammation of the throat, this pair is favorably combined with Shan Dou Gen (Radix Sophorae Subprostratae), Ban Lan Gen (Radix Isatidis Seu Baphicacanthi), and Xuan Shen (Radix Scrophulariae Ningpoensis).

Comments:

(a) Pu Gong Ying and Zi Hua Di Ding along with Ye Ju Hua (Flos Chrysanthemi Indici), which is less powerful than the first two medicinals, are the more effective Chinese medicinals for the treatment of dermatological problems due to heat toxins.

(b) It should be noted that Pu Gong Ying is also called Huang Hua Di Ding, yellow flowered Di Ding. Zi Hua Di Ding is the purple flowered Di Ding.

Pu Huang (Pollen Typhae) & Wu Ling Zhi (Feces Trogopterori Seu Pteromi)

Individual properties:	
Pu Huang	**Wu Ling Zhi**
Cools the blood and stops bleeding by astringing Quickens the blood and dispels stasis Superior for stopping bleeding Better for treating pain due to blood stasis of the heat type Usual dosage: 6-10g	Quickens the blood and dispels stasis, stops bleeding by dispelling stasis Moves the qi and stops pain Superior for stopping pain Better for treating pain due to blood stasis of the cold type Usual dosage: 6-12g

Properties when combined:

When these two medicinals are combined together, they effectively quicken the blood, dispel stasis, and stop pain.

Major indications of the combination:

1. Epigastric, cardiac, abdominal, and lateral costal pain due to qi stagnation and blood stasis (1) (2)
2. Menstrual irregularities, amenorrhea, dysmenorrhea, postpartum abdominal pain, and retention of the lochia due to blood stasis (1) (3)

Notes:

(1) For these indications, this combination is used in *Shi Xiao San* (Loose a Smile Powder).[6]

(2) For these indications, uncooked *Pu Huang* and vinegar mix-fried *Wu Ling Zhi* should be prescribed.

(3) For these indications, uncooked *Pu Huang* and wine mix-fried *Wu Ling Zhi* should be prescribed.

Comment:

(a) The pair *Pu Huang* and *Wu Ling Zhi* which makes up *Shi Xiao San* can serve as a basic treatment for numerous disorders where pain is the main complaint: In case of gynecological disorders due to qi stagnation and blood stasis, it is useful to add *Dang Gui* (Radix Angelicae Sinensis), *Chuan Xiong* (Radix Ligustici Wallichii), and *Xiang Fu* (Rhizoma Cyperi Rotundi) to *Shi Xiao San*. In case of abdominal or epigastric pain due to blood stasis and cold, add *Gan Jiang* (dry Rhizoma Zingiberis) and *Gao Liang Jiang* (Rhizoma Alpiniae Officinari) to *Shi Xiao San*. In case of cardiac pain due to blood stasis, it is useful to add *Dan Shen* (Radix Salviae Miltiorrhizae), *San Qi* (Radix Pseudoginseng), and *Tan Xiang* (Lignum Santali Albi). For postpartum abdominal pain with retention of the lochia due to blood stasis, add *Chuan Niu Xi* (Radix Cyathulae Officinalis), *Yi Mu Cao* (Herba Leonuris Heterophylli), *San Qi* (Radix Pseudoginseng), and *Shan Zha* (Fructus Crataegi). For lateral costal pain due to blood stasis, add *Yan Hu Suo* (Rhizoma Corydalis Yanhusuo), *Yu Jin* (Tuber Curcumae), and *Chuan Xiong* (Radix Ligustici Wallichii).

---

[6] Bensky & Barolet, in their *Chinese Herbal Medicine: Formulas & Strategies*, Eastland Press, Seattle, call this formula Sudden Smile Powder. The word *shi* means to lose. Because the patient is freed from pain after taking this formula, they let loose a smile.

Sang Ji Sheng (Ramulus Loranthi Seu Visci) & Sang Zhi (Ramulus Mori Albi)

Individual properties:	
Sang Ji Sheng	**Sang Zhi**
Supplements the liver & kidneys Strengthens the sinews, bones, and lumbus Supplements the blood and nourishes the vessels Dispels wind dampness Usual dosage: 10-30g	Frees the four limbs and disinhibits the joints Frees the flow of the channels and stops pain Dispels wind, dampness, and heat Usual dosage: 15-30g

Properties when combined:

One supplements; the other dispels.
One nourishes; the other frees the flow.
When these medicinals are combined together, they supplement the liver and kidneys, strengthen the sinews and bones, dispel wind dampness, free the flow of the network vessels and stop pain.

Major indications of the combination:

1. Low back and limb pain, numbness of the limbs, loss of joint mobility, and rheumatic pain due to wind damp *bi* and kidney or blood vacuity in turn due to malnourishment of the sinews

2. Arterial hypertension with headache, vertigo, tinnitus, and heart palpitations due to liver-kidney yin vacuity causing liver yang hyperactivity

Comment:

(a) *Sang Ji Sheng* has been shown to be effective in the treatment of arterial hypertension, hypercholesterolemia, and coronary heart disease at dosages of 30-60g per day. It is especially effective when these disorders are caused by ascendant hyperactivity of liver yang due to liver-kidney yin vacuity.

Sha Ren (Fructus Amomi) & Shu Di (Cooked Radix Rehmanniae)

Individual properties:	
Sha Ren	**Shu Di**
Moves the qi and rectifies the middle burner Transforms dampness and warms the middle burner Arouses the spleen and stimulates the appetite Guides the qi towards the kidneys Usual dosage: 2-5g	Supplements the blood and nourishes fluids and humors Nourishes the liver and enriches the kidneys Slimy and rich in nature, difficult to assimilate, tends to block the stomach qi Usual dosage: 10-30g

Properties when combined:

When these two medicinals are combined together, they strongly nourish the blood, essence, and yin without giving rise to qi stagnation or loss of appetite.

Major indications of the combination:

1. Liver-kidney yin or essence vacuity, blood vacuity associated with weakness of the spleen and stomach, particularly due to loss of control over their movement and transformation functions (1)

Note:

(1) In this case, *Sha Ren Ban Shu Di* is prescribed or, in other words, *Shu Di* mixed with seeds of *Sha Ren*. *Sha Ren Ke*, the shell of *Amomum Villosum*, can also be used if spleen vacuity is not pronounced.

Comments:

(a) *Sha Ren* focuses the action of *Shu Di* on the kidneys.

(b) The seeds of *Sha Ren* should be crushed before decoction and added not more than 10 minutes before the end of the cooking.

Sheng Di (Uncooked Radix Rehmanniae) & *Shi Gao* (Gypsum Fibrosum)

Individual properties:	
Sheng Di	***Shi Gao***
Goes towards the blood division Cools the blood and stops bleeding Nourishes yin and clears heat Clears heart fire Usual dosage: 15-30g	Goes towards the qi division Clears *yang ming* & qi division heat Drains lung & stomach heat Usual dosage: 15-60g

Properties when combined:

One is for the blood division; the other is for the qi division.
When these two medicinals are combined together, they clear heat from the qi and blood divisions.

Major indications of the combination:

1. High fever, great thirst, eruption of reddish macula, hemorrhage, mental confusion, a red tongue, and scarlet, dry lips due to heat in qi and blood divisions (1)
2. Bleeding gums, gingivitis, oral ulcers, toothache, and thirst due to stomach heat damaging kidney yin (2)

Notes:

(1) For these indications, this combination is used in *Qing Wen Bai Du Yin* (Clear Warmth & Vanquish Toxins Drink).

(2) For these indications, this combination is included in *Yu Nu Jian* (Jade Maiden Decoction). Traditionally, it is *Shu Di* which is used in this formula. However, to clear stomach heat more strongly, *Shu Di* is frequently replaced by *Sheng Di*.

Comments:

(a) For the side effects of *Sheng Di*, see comment (d) from the pair *Sheng Di* and *Shu Di* below.

(b) For food incompatibilities of *Sheng Di*, see comment (b) of the pair *Sheng Di* and *Shu Di* below.

Sheng Di (Uncooked Radix Rehmanniae) & Shu Di (Cooked Radix Rehmanniae)

Individual properties:	
Sheng Di	**Shu Di**
Clears heat and cools the blood Enriches yin, engenders fluids, and nourishes the blood Usual dosage: 10-15g	Supplements blood & yin Nourishes the liver & kidneys Boosts the essence and fills the bone marrow Usual dosage: 10-30g

Properties when combined:

When these two medicinals are combined together, they mutually reinforce each other. Together, they enrich liver-kidney yin, boost the essence and fill the bone marrow, supplement the blood and engender fluids, cool the blood and clear heat.

Major indications of the combination:

1. Persistent, low-grade fever due to warm disease damaging yin (fluids)
2. Tidal fever and steaming bones due to yin (essence) vacuity or blood vacuity
3. Vertigo, insomnia, menstrual irregularities, oligomenorrhea, and metrorrhagia due to liver-kidney blood and essence vacuity

Note:

(1) For these indications, this combination is used in *Er Huang San* (Two Yellows Powder).

Comments:

(a) In clinical practice, when writing a prescription, this combination is called *Er Di*, the two *Di* or *Sheng Shu Di*, uncooked & cooked *Di*.

(b) *Sheng Di* and *Shu Di* are incompatible with blood from any type of animal, onions, chives, turnips, kohlrabi, radishes, and garlic.

(c) This combination is very rich, slimy, and difficult to digest. To avoid any qi stagnation and in case of spleen weakness, it is useful to add *Sha Ren* (Fructus Amomi). See note (1) of the pair *Sha Ren* and *Shu Di* above.

(d) The use of *Sheng Di* in the beginning of treatment can sometimes cause diarrhea or loose stools for 1-3 days. Most of the time, this diarrhea stops by itself. If it continues, the dosage should be diminished and *Sha Ren* should be added. Sometimes, treatment must even be discontinued.

Sheng Di (Uncooked Radix Rehmanniae) & Xi Xin (Herba Asari Cum Radice)

Individual properties:	
Sheng Di	**Xi Xin**
Clears heat and cools the blood Enriches yin and engenders fluids Nourishes the blood Stops bleeding Usual dosage: 6-10g	Dispels wind cold Warms the interior Dispels wind and stops pain Frees the flow of the network vessels and stops pain Dosage: 1-3g

Properties when combined:

When these two medicinals are combined together, *Xi Xin,* which is acrid, dispelling, and upbearing, carries *Sheng Di,* which is sweet, cold, and clearing, towards the upper burner to clear heat. Together, they dispel wind, clear heat, and stop pain without drying.

Major indications of the combination:

1. Headache and toothache due to wind fire or vacuity fire (1)

Note:

(1) The combination of *Xi Xin* and *Shi Gao* (Gypsum Fibrosum) also treats headaches, toothache, and oral ulcers. However, the causes of these disorders for which *Xi Xin* and *Shi Gao* are effective are different from those for which *Sheng Di* and *Shi Gao* are indicated. *Xi Xin* and *Shi Gao* act on stomach fire, while *Sheng Di* and *Xi Xin* act more on wind heat or vacuity heat.

Comments:

(a) It should be noted that *Xi Xin* is a powerful analgesic, notably when the pain is located in the head, teeth, bones, nose, and mouth. Despite the fact that *Xi Xin* is warming and dispelling in nature and, therefore, particularly adapted to wind cold, it can also be used for any type of pattern in order to benefit from its analgesic action if it is combined with other medicinals which are appropriate for the pattern.

(b) One should be careful with the dosage of *Xi Xin.* It can become toxic beginning at as little as 5g per day. As the ancient saying goes, "(For) *Xi Xin,* do not exceed a *qian.*" (One *qian* equals approximately 3g.) Therefore, one should not exceed 3g of *Xi Xin* per day and closely observe the patient's reactions. The most common signs of Asarum intoxication are headache, vertigo, perspiration, rapid breathing, chest oppression, abnormal dilation of the pupils, a warm body, arterial hypertension, etc. As long as the proper dosage is respected, such manifestations are otherwise rarely seen.

Sheng Jiang (Uncooked Rhizoma Zingiberis) & Zhu Ru (Caulis Bambusae In Taeniis)

Individual properties:	
Sheng Jiang	*Zhu Ru*
Warms the middle burner and transforms phlegm Harmonizes the stomach and drains cold, downbears counterflow and stops vomiting Usual dosage: 3-10g	Clears heat and transforms phlegm Harmonizes the stomach and clears the stomach, downbears counterflow and stops vomiting Usual dosage: 3-10g

Properties when combined:

One is warm; the other is cold.
When these two medicinals are combined together, they effectively harmonize the stomach and downbear stomach qi counterflow, transform phlegm accumulated in the middle burner, eliminate cold and heat, and stop vomiting.

Major indications of the combination:

1. Nausea, vomiting, and hiccup due to stomach disharmony and stomach qi counterflow due to mixed cold and heat in the stomach or accumulation of phlegm in the stomach

Comment:

(a) This pair forms one of the most powerful combinations to stop vomiting. *Sheng Jiang* is renowned as being "an essential medicinal for vomiting" and *Zhu Ru* is one of the best Chinese medicinals for vomiting due to stomach heat or stomach accumulation of phlegm heat.

Shi Chang Pu (Rhizoma Acori Graminei) & Yuan Zhi (Radix Polygalae Tenuifoliae)

Individual properties:	
Shi Chang Pu	*Yuan Zhi*
Opens the orifices or portals of the heart Transforms phlegm confounding the portals of the heart Rectifies the qi and transforms phlegm Arouses & quiets the spirit Usual dosage: 3-10g	Re-establishes the interaction between the heart & kidneys Supplements the heart qi Quiets the spirit and boosts the intelligence Transforms phlegm and opens the orifices Usual dosage: 6-10g

Properties when combined:

When these two medicinals are combined together, they go to the heart, transform phlegm, and open the portals of the heart. They re-establish the interaction between the heart and kidneys, boost the intelligence, and arouse the spirit.

Major indications of the combination:

1. Mental confusion, mental retardation, decrease of intellectual acuity, vertigo, insomnia, and mental agitation due to heart and kidneys not interacting or phlegm confounding the orifices of the heart (1) (2)

Notes:

(1) This combination is used in *Yuan Zhi Tang* (Polygala Decoction), *Zhen Zhong Dan* (Pillow Elixir), and *Sang Piao Xiao San* (Mantis Egg Case Powder).

(2) *Yuan Zhi, i.e.,* uncooked *Yuan Zhi,* is irritating to the gastric mucous membranes and produces nausea and vomiting. That is the reason why *Yuan Zhi* is contraindicated in case of gastritis or gastric ulcers and why licorice-processed *Yuan Zhi* or honey mix-fried *Yuan Zhi* are systematically prescribed.

Comments:

(a) Together, *Shi Chuang Pu, Yuan Zhi* ,and *Fu Shen* (Sclerotium Pararadicis Poriae Cocos), which are used together, for example, in *Sang Piao Xiao San,* have the property of re-establishing the interaction between the heart and kidneys. While *Shi Chang Pu* opens the orifices of the heart, *Yuan Zhi* moves the kidney qi, and *Fu Shen* downbears heart qi toward the kidneys. Along with the pairs, *Huang Lian* and *E Jiao* and *Huang Lian* and *Rou Gui,* they are the most effective Chinese medicinals for re-establishing the interaction between the heart and kidneys.

(b) For the differences between *Shi Chang Pu, Jiu Jie Chang Pu, Xian Chang Pu,* and *Shui Chang Pu,* see comment (a) of the pair *Ci Shi* and *Shi Chang Pu.*

(c) *Shi Chang Pu* is incompatible with blood and mutton as well as Maltose (*Yi Tang*).

Shi Gao (Gypsum Fibrosum) & *Xi Xin* (Herba Asari Cum Radice)

Individual properties:	
Shi Gao	**Xi Xin**
Sweet, very cold, heavy, draining, downbearing Clears heat and drains fire Resolves the muscle aspect Eliminates vexation Drains stomach & lung heat Usual dosage: 15-30g	Acrid, warm, light, dispelling, upbearing Dispels wind cold Dispels floating heat from the orifices of the upper burner Frees the flow of the network vessels and stops the pain Usual dosage: 1-3g

Properties when combined:

One is cold; the other is hot. Thus their opposite natures combine and complement each other. *Xi Xin,* acrid, dispelling, and upbearing, carries *Shi Gao,* cold, clearing, and draining, towards the upper burner to clear heat.
When these two medicinals are combined together, they clear heat and drain fire, free the flow of the network vessels and stop pain.

Major indications of the combination:

1. Toothache, bleeding gums, swollen, painful gums, oral ulcers, and glossitis due to stagnation of heat in the stomach
2. Headache due to wind heat entering the clear orifices

Comments:

(a) *Xi Xin*'s tropism is markedly towards the mouth, tongue, teeth, and gums. This medicinal treats pain and inflammations in this area. *Xi Xin* guides the action of *Shi Gao* towards the upper burner due to its upbearing nature.

(b) Despite the fact that it has a very pronounced warm nature, *Xi Xin* may be used, in combination with other medicinal substances, for all types of patterns — repletion or vacuity, cold or heat, internal or external — in order to benefit from its remarkable analgesic effects.

(c) For precautions in the use of *Xi Xin,* see comment (d) from the pair *Sheng Di* and *Xi Xin.*

Shi Gao (Gypsum Fibrosum) & Zhi Mu (Rhizoma Anemarrhenae Aspheloidis)

Individual properties:	
Shi Gao	**Zhi Mu**
Sweet, acrid, cold Heavy body and downbearing property Clears replete heat from the qi division and *yang ming* channels Clears heat from the lungs & stomach Only treats replete heat Usual dosage: 15-30g	Bitter, sweet, cold, moistening Rich body and moistening property Nourishes yin, moistens dryness, and drains ministerial fire Clears heat from the lungs & stomach Treats replete & vacuity heat Usual dosage: 6-10g

Properties when combined:

One tends to clear; the other to moisten. When these two medicinals are combined together, they strongly clear and drain replete heat while protecting fluids and yin. Together, they effectively clear replete heat from the lungs and stomach.

Major indications of the combination:

1. Persistent high fever, great thirst and desire for cold drinks, a dry tongue, vexation, profuse perspiration, and a surging, big pulse due to heat in the qi division (1)
2. Upper thirsting & wasting with polydipsia, a dry mouth and tongue, and great thirst due to replete lung heat damaging fluids (2)

Notes:

(1) For these indications, this combination is used in *Bai Hu Tang* (White Tiger Decoction). For these indications, uncooked *Shi Gao* and uncooked *Zhi Mu* should be prescribed.

(2) For these indications, uncooked *Shi Gao* and stir-fried *Zhi Mu* should be prescribed.

Comments:

(a) *Shi Gao* and *Zhi Mu* are the essential elements of the therapeutic action of *Bai Hu Tang* since the other two medicinals, *Gan Cao* (Radix Glycyrrhizae) and *Geng Mi* (Semen Oryzae Sativae), are mainly used to soften the drastic action of this pair and protect the stomach.

(b) "The four major symptoms" or "the big four" are the specific signs and symptoms of the pattern of heat in the *yang ming* channels and heat in the qi division which *Bai Hu Tang* and, thus, the pair *Shi Gao* and *Zhi Mu* specifically treat. The four big symptoms are 1) high fever, 2) profuse perspiration, 3) great thirst, and 4) a surging pulse. However, high fever is the central symptom of the pattern. The intense internal heat expels the liquids towards the exterior, causing profuse perspiration. The loss of fluids then causes great thirst. The heat surges upward internally, dilating the vessels, and qi accumulates which causes the blood to gush in the vessels. Hence the pulse becomes big and surging.

(c) According to Wu Ju-tong's *Wen Bing Tiao Bian (The Methodological Discrimination of Warm Diseases)*, "the four prohibitions"[7]

---

7   Wiseman gives contraindication for *jiu*. However, this is a modern Western medical term. In terms of the premodern Western medical literature, we believe the straight forward translation of prohibition is closer in meaning and tone to the Chinese. Inevitably, there are problems when a single word is used in both a traditional Chinese medical sense and a modern Western medical sense.

correspond to *Bai Hu Tang*'s "four big" (indications). These four prohibitions are: 1) a floating, wiry, fine pulse, 2) a deep pulse, 3) no thirst, and 4) no perspiration.

A floating pulse means that the external evils are located on the exterior. *Bai Hu Tang* treats internal heat. Therefore, the use of *Bai Hu Tang* is prohibited if there is a floating pulse. A wiry, fine pulse often means a disorder of the liver and, in particular, a liver blood or yin vacuity. *Bai Hu Tang* treats repletion, not vacuity. Therefore, if there is a wiry, fine pulse, *Bai Hu Tang* is prohibited.

A deep pulse means that the condition is an internal disease. If the pulse is deep and without force, it indicates an internal vacuity. *Bai Hu Tang* treats repletion, not vacuity. If the pulse is deep and forceful, this indicates (internal) heat accumulated in the *yang ming* bowels. The therapeutic principles in that case are to discharge heat accumulated in the stomach and intestines by precipitating, as with *Da Cheng Qi Tang* (Major Order the Qi Decoction). Since *Bai Hu Tang* categorically treats heat located in the *yang ming* channel (and not in the *yang ming* bowels, its treatment principles are to clear heat and drain fire from the *yang ming* channel and not precipitating heat through defecation. Therefore, a deep, forceless or deep, forceful pulse prohibit the use *Bai Hu Tang*.

The absence of thirst together with fever can be found in damage due to wind cold sometimes in light wind heat, heat in the blood division, and in damp heat patterns. *Bai Hu Tang* does not treat any of these imbalances. Therefore, absence of thirst prohibits the prescribing of *Bai Hu Tang*.

The absence of perspiration together with fever can be found in several patterns, such as wind cold of the repletion type where cold blocks the pores of the skin and some warm diseases where fluids have been so wasted that there are not enough fluids left to produce perspiration. Because *Bai Hu Tang* categorically does not treat in any instance these imbalances, absence of perspiration prohibits or contraindicates its prescription.

(d) It is cold-natured and bitter-tasting medicinals which ordinarily clear heat and drain fire. Therefore, why use *Shi Gao* and *Zhi Mu* to clear the qi division? Why not use medicinals such as *Huang Lian* (Rhizoma Coptidis Chinensis), *Huang Qin* (Radix Scutellariae Baicalensis), and *Zhi Zi* (Fructus Gardeniae Jasminoidis)? When heat invades the qi division, it causes profuse perspiration. This damages yin. The treatment principle then consists of using cold medicinals to clear heat but also sweet ones to moisten. Sweet and cold tend to moisten dryness and enrich yin, as in the case of *Shi Gao*. The cold nature and the bitter taste of *Huang Lian*, *Huang Qin*, and *Zhi Zi* drain heat effectively. However, the bitter taste also tends to dry dampness and thus damage yin. In the present case, yin is already threatened by heat. Accentuation of this tendency should, therefore, be avoided.

If bitter damages yin, why use *Zhi Mu* which is bitter? First, the bitterness of *Zhi Mu* is much less powerful than that of *Huang Lian* or *Zhi Zi*. Moreover, *Zhi Mu* is moistening and nourishes yin. This allows this medicinal to drain fire (bitter, cold) without drying (moistening property). To the contrary, it actually engenders fluids.

Shi Gao (Gypsum Fibrosum) & *Zhu Ye* (Folium Bambusae)

Individual properties:	
Shi Gao	***Zhu Ye***
Acrid, sweet, very cold Heavy, downbearing, draining Drains fire and clears the qi division Clears lung & stomach heat Eliminates vexation and stops thirst Usual dosage: 15-60g	Acrid, sweet, cold Light, floating, dispelling Dispels wind heat, clears the defensive Clears heat from the lungs & heart Eliminates vexation and stops thirst Usual dosage: 5-15g

Properties when combined:

One is heavy, while the other is light.
One is downbearing; the other is upbearing.
One is draining; the other is dispelling.
When these two medicinals are combined together, they clear heat in the upper and lower parts of the body as well as in both the interior and exterior. Together they effectively clear heat in the lungs, stomach, and heart, eliminate vexation and stop thirst.

Major indications of the combination:

1. Persistent fever due to retained heat in the lungs and stomach damaging the qi and yin, as in the terminal phase of a warm disease, with vexatious heat, chest oppression, nausea, vomiting, and thirst (1)
2. Cough, a sensation of heat in the chest, and thirst due to heat in the lungs
3. Glossitis, oral ulcers, stomatitis, foul breath, and thirst due to stomach heat

Note:

(1) For these indications, this combination is used in *Zhu Ye Shi Gao Tang* (Bamboo & Gypsum Decoction).

Comments:

(a) *Zhu Ye*, *Zhu Ye Juan Xin*, and *Dan Zhu Ye* are three different medicinals. It is important to distinguish them in order to prescribe them correctly. *Zhu Ye* is the mature leaf of *Phyllostachys nigra*. *Zhu Ye Juan Xin* is the young, tender leaf of *Phyllostachys nigra* which is starting to grow but which is still rolled up. *Dan Zhu Ye* is the upper part of the stem with the inflorescence of *Lophatherum gracile*. *Zhu Ye*, *Zhu Ye Juan Xin*, and *Dan Zhu* all clear heat, eliminate vexation, and disinhibit urination. However, *Zhu Ye* is superior for dispelling wind heat and superior for clearing heat. It is used for thirst and vexation due to a warm disease damaging qi and yin. *Zhu Ye Juan Xin* is superior for clearing the heart and eliminating vexation. It is mainly used for mental confusion, delirium, loss of consciousness, and vexation due to heat attacking the pericardium. *Dan Zhu Ye* is superior for clearing and eliminating damp heat, promoting diuresis, and clearing heart heat transmitted to the small intestine. It is used for jaundice, dysuria, and oliguria due to damp heat or heart fire being transmitted to the small intestine.

(b) *Shi Gao* stops thirst not by engendering fluids directly (like *Lu Gen* [Rhizoma Phragmitis Communis] or *Ge Gen* [Radix Puerariae]), but by clearing heat which damages fluids and causes thirst.

(c) To obtain the maximum effectiveness from *Shi Gao*, its powdered form should be used when preparing the decoction.

Tao Ren (Semen Pruni Persicae) & *Xing Ren* (Semen Pruni Armeniacae)

Individual properties:	
Tao Ren	**Xing Ren**
Oleaginous seed from the peach Moistens dryness and lubricates the intestines Quickens the blood, dispels stasis, stops pain Treats constipation due to large intestine fluid dryness Usual dosage: 6-10g	Oleaginous seed from the apricot Moistens the intestines and frees the flow of the stools Quickens the blood and downbears the qi Eliminates phlegm and stops cough Treats constipation due to qi stagnation and dryness Usual dosage: 6-10g

Properties when combined:

One is for the blood division; the other is for the qi division.
When these two medicinals are combined together, they quicken the blood, move the qi, and stop pain, moisten the intestines and free the flow of the stools.

Major indications of the combination:

1. Chest, epigastric, and lower abdominal pain due to qi stagnation and blood stasis (1)
2. Constipation of the vacuity type due to dryness in the large intestine (2) (3)
3. Constipation of the repletion type due to qi stagnation (3)

Notes:

(1) For these indications, uncooked *Tao Ren* and uncooked *Xing Ren* should be prescribed.

(2) For these indications, this combination is used in *Wu Ren Wan* (Five Seeds Pills).

(3) For these indications, stir-fried till yellow *Tao Ren* and uncooked *Xing Ren* should be prescribed.

Comments:

(a) Regarding the toxicity of *Tao Ren* and *Xing Ren*, see respectively comment (a) of the pair *Hong Hua* and *Tao Ren* and comment (d) of the pair *Chuan Bei Mu* and *Xing Ren* above.

(b) *Huo Ma Ren* (Semen Cannabis Sativae) is very effective for treating constipation but is forbidden in many Western countries. In many cases, it can be replaced by *Tao Ren* for moistening the intestines and freeing the flow of the stools.

Wu Wei Zi (Fructus Schisandrae Chinensis) & Xi Xin (Herba Asari Cum Radice)

Individual properties:	
Wu Wei Zi	**Xi Xin**
Sour, astringent, secures and holds Constrains the lung qi and nourishes the kidneys Engenders fluids Stops perspiration Secures the essence and stops diarrhea Usual dosage: 3-10g	Acrid, dispelling, warm, frees the flow Warms the lungs and transforms phlegm Scatters cold and resolves the exterior Expels wind and stops pain Opens the nose orifices Usual dosage: 1-3g

Properties when combined:

One is sour and astringing; the other is acrid and dispelling.
One constrains; the other opens.
When these two medicinals are combined together, they complement each other and combine the methods of diffusion and constraint. Together, they effectively transform phlegm and diffuse the lung qi, constrain the lung qi, stop cough and calm asthma.

Major indications of the combination:

1. Cough and asthma due to wind cold and/or accumulation of phlegm cold in the lungs (1) (2)
2. Chronic cough and asthma due to lung-kidney vacuity (3)

Notes:

(1) For these indications, this combination is used in *Xiao Qing Long Tang* (Minor Blue Dragon Decoction) and *Wu Wei Xi Xin Tang* (Schisandra & Asarum Decoction).

(2) In this case, dispelling, diffusing, and opening are the priorities. Therefore, the dosage of *Xi Xin* should be relatively greater than for *Wu Wei Zi*.

(3) In this case the objective is more to constrain lung qi and nourish the kidneys. Therefore, the dosage for *Wu Wei Zi* should be relatively larger than for *Xi Xin*.

Comments:

(a) The lungs govern the qi and breathing, downbear and diffuse the qi. When there is a wind cold attack, the lung qi is blocked by the external evils and diffusion and downbearing of the qi is disturbed. In this case, the treatment principles consist of dispelling wind cold and warming and diffusing the lungs. This is the role of *Xi Xin*. In case of cough, lung qi is counterflowing and rises against the normal flow. If the affection is not resolved, it tends to damage the lung qi. In that case, the treatment principles consist of rectifying and constraining the lung qi. This is the role of *Wu Wei Zi*. If cough is due to an external agent, *Wu Wei Zi* only treats the branch manifestation, *i.e.*, the counterflowing qi. If it is due to lung-kidney vacuity, *Wu Wei Zi* treats the branch manifestation, *i.e.*, the counterflowing qi, *and* the root cause, *i.e.*, lung-kidney vacuity.

(b) *Xi Xin* is upbearing, floating, and diffuses the lung qi. *Wu Wei Zi* is astringent, sinking, and constrains the lung qi. How can these two medicinals with such opposite affects on the qi be combined in the treatment of cough? In fact, this opposition is only a seeming contradiction. *Xi Xin* reinforces the natural (physiological) movement of qi of the lungs — diffusion. When a pathological agent blocks the diffusing function of the lungs (floating movement), *Xi Xin* frees the flow of the lung qi and promotes its floating movement. *Wu Wei Zi* inhibits and is opposed to a *pathological* movement of lung qi, *i.e.*, lung qi counterflow. Contrary to the effect of a medicinal like *Xing Ren* (Semen Pruni Armeniacae) which downbears qi that is already counterflowing, *Wu Wei Zi* prevents the lung qi from rising by holding it down near its source. In other words, *Xi Xin* promotes normal physiological movement, while *Wu Wei Zi* prevents pathological movement. *Xi Xin* regulates the diffusion of the lung qi; *Wu Wei Zi* regulates the descent of lung qi. This is why these two medicinals do not contradict each other and function well together.

© There are two types of *Wu Wei Zi*. *Bei Wu Wei Zi* (northern *Wu Wei Zi, Schisandra Chinensis* Baill.) is astringent. Therefore, it constrains the lung qi, stops perspiration, secures the essence, and stops diarrhea. It also tends to supplement the heart, lungs, and kidneys. It is clinically the most prescribed type of *Wu Wei Zi*. It is used, for example, in *Du Qi Wan* (Prosperous Qi Pills). *Nan Wu Wei Zi* (southern *Wu Wei Zi, Schisandra splenanthera* Rehd. et Wils.) tends to rectify the qi, transform dampness, and disperse phlegm. It treats cough or asthma due to wind cold and/or an accumulation of phlegm. It has no supplementing property. It is used, for example, in *Xiao Qing Long Tang* (Minor Blue Dragon Decoction).

Wu Yao (Radix Linderae Strychnifoliae) & *Yan Hu Suo* (Rhizoma Corydalis Yanhusuo)

Individual properties:	
Wu Yao	**Yan Hu Suo**
Tropism: the qi division Moves the qi and stops pain Warms & scatters cold in the liver & kidney channels Stops pain, particularly in the epigastric and lower abdominal areas Usual dosage: 3-10g	Tropism: the blood division Quickens the blood and moves the qi Stops pain efficiently Stops pain in the whole body — the upper & lower, interior & exterior Usual dosage: 3-10g

Properties when combined:

One rectifies the qi; the other the blood. When these two medicinals are combined together, they effectively quicken the blood and dispel stasis, move the qi and stop pain.

Major indications of the combination:

1. Epigastric and abdominal pain due to qi stagnation and blood stasis (1)
2. Inguinal hernia and scrotal pain and distention (*i.e., shan*) due to qi and cold stagnation in the liver and kidney channels (2)

Notes:

(1) For these indications, wine mix-fried *Wu Yao* and wine mix-fried *Yan Hu Suo* should be prescribed.

(2) For these indications, salt mix-fried *Wu Yao* and vinegar mix-fried *Yan Hu Suo* should be prescribed.

Comments:

(a) *Yan Hu Suo* is a medicinal for the qi within the blood. This is to say that it moves the yang aspect of the blood. Moreover, it is said that it disperses qi stagnation in the blood and blood stasis in the qi. It is, therefore, a medicinal which quickens simultaneously the qi and blood, but which, nevertheless, has more of an action on the blood.

(b) *Wu Yao's* area of pronounced action is the abdomen in general and the lower abdomen in particular. Therefore, *Wu Yao* guides the action of *Yan Hu Suo* to the abdomen in general and especially to the lower abdomen.

(c) *Yan Hu Suo* is one of the major pain-stopping medicinals in the whole Chinese materia medica.

It is prescribed in all types of patterns whenever pain is a dominant symptom.

(d) For the definition of *shan*, see note (1) of the pair *Ju He* and *Li Zhi He* above.

Xiang Fu (Rhizoma Cyperi Rotundi) & *Yi Mu Cao* (Herba Leonuri Heterophylli)

Individual properties:	
Xiang Fu	**Yi Mu Cao**
Tropism: the qi division but also the blood Drains the liver and resolves depression Harmonizes the qi & blood, moves the qi to quicken the blood, regulates the menses Usual dosage: 3-10g	Tropism: the blood division Quickens the blood and regulates the menses Dispels stasis without damaging the blood Nourishes the blood without engendering stasis Usual dosage: 15-30g

Properties when combined:

One is for the qi; the other is for the blood. These are two key medicinals for gynecological problems.
When these two medicinals are combined together, they effectively move the qi and resolve depression, quicken the blood and dispel stasis, and regulate the menses.

Major indications of the combination:

1. Menstrual irregularities, abdominal pain and distention before the period, postpartum abdominal pain, and dysmenorrhea due to qi stagnation (liver) and blood stasis (1)
2. Traumatic injury

Note:

(1) For these indications, vinegar mix-fried *Xiang Fu* and wine mix-fried *Yi Mu Cao* should be prescribed.

Comments:

(a) *Xiang Fu* has a pronounced tropism for gynecological disorders. Women belong to blood and tend to suffer easily from blood imbalances. *Xiang Fu* is a medicinal for the blood within the qi since it tends to rectify the blood by rectifying the qi.

(b) *Yi Mu Cao* only slightly nourishes the blood and cannot be used by itself to nourish the blood. It must be combined with other, more powerful medicinals for nourishing the blood, like *Dang Gui* (Radix Angelicae Sinensis) or *Shu Di* (cooked Radix Rehmanniae).

(c) *Yi Mu Cao* means the plant (*cao*) which boosts or benefits (*yi*) the mother (*mu*). *Yi Mu Cao* is a key medicinal for numerous gynecological disorders and is particularly effective for easing labor. However, *Yi Mu Cao* is only effective at a relatively high dosage, *i.e.*, 15-30g generally. It may even be prescribed up to 100g in severe cases or for delivery.

Yu Jin (Tuber Curcumae) & Zhi Ke (Fructus Immaturus Citri Aurantii)

Individual properties:	
Yu Jin	**Zhi Ke**
Tropism: the blood & qi divisions Dispels stasis and stops pain Moves the qi and resolves liver depression Disinhibits the gallbladder and treats jaundice Usual dosage: 9-15g	Tropism: the qi division Moves the qi and disperses distention Loosens the chest & diaphragm Disperses food accumulation Usual dosage: 5-10g

Properties when combined:

One is for the blood division; the other for the qi division.
When these two medicinals are combined together, they complement each other. Together, they effectively move the qi and quicken the blood, resolve depression and stop pain.

Major indications of the combination:

1. Piercing pain and distention in the lateral costal region due to liver depression qi stagnation causing liver blood stasis (1)
2. Pain and distention of the epigastrium and lateral costal region due to liver-stomach disharmony with qi stagnation which progressively produces blood stasis (1)

Note:

(1) For these indications, vinegar mix-fried *Yu Jin* and uncooked *Zhi Ke* should be prescribed.

Comments:

(a) There are two types of *Yu Jin. Guan Yu Yin* comes mainly from Sichuan province. It is also called *Huang Yu Jin* or yellow *Yu Jin*. Acrid, bitter, and fragrant, it tends to be directed towards the qi division. Mainly, it moves the qi and resolves depression. Secondarily, it quickens the blood. *Chuan Yu Jin* comes mainly from Zhejiang province. It is also called *Hei Yu Jin*, black *Yu Jin*. Acrid, bland, and cool, it tends to be directed towards the blood division. Mainly, it quickens the blood, dispels stasis, and stops pain. Secondarily, it rectifies the qi.

(b) *Zhi Ke* and *Zhi Shi* (Fructus Citri Aurantii) both come from *Citrus Aurantium. Zhi Ke* is the big, ripe fruit. Therefore, it is also called *Da Zhi Ke. Zhi Shi* is the small, immature fruit. Therefore, it is also called *Xiao Zhi Shi. Zhi Ke* and *Zhi Shi* have similar actions, but *Zhi Shi* is more powerful and *Zhi Ke* is more moderate. Thus, *Zhi Ke* disperses the qi, while *Zhi Shi* breaks the qi. If qi stagnation is severe, *Zhi Shi* should be prescribed. If it is moderate or if it is accompanied by vacuity, *Zhi Ke* should be prescribed.

Glossary of formulas not appearing in *Formulas & Strategies*

The overwhelming majority of formulas mentioned in this book are included in Bensky & Barolet's *Chinese Herbal Medicine: Formulas & Strategies*, Eastland Press, Seattle, 1990. This is the most common standard reference on Chinese medicinal formulas in English. Therefore, below, the reader will find the ingredients of only those formulas mentioned in the text which do not appear in *Formulas & Strategies*.

All of the dosages of the following formulas are given as a) daily dosages for making decoctions from the whole or bulk-dispensed medicinals, b) in grams, and c) for adults. These dosages are only suggestive and should be adapted for individual patients based on one's understanding of prescribing Chinese medicinals and taking into account the patient's sex, age, weight, constitution, and nature of their complaint and the season of the year. Those practitioners prescribing Chinese medicinals as desiccated powdered extracts should follow the guidelines of the manufacturers of those extracts for converting these dosages into the appropriate dosages for such powdered extracts.

Bai He Zhi Mu Tang (Lily & Anemarrhena Decoction): *Bai He* (Bulbus Lilii), 15g, *Zhi Mu* (Rhizoma Anemarrhenae Aspheloidis), 12g

Bai Zhu San [1] (Atractylodes Powder): *Bai Zhu* (Rhizoma Atractylodis Macrocephalae), 15g, *Fu Ling* (Sclerotium Poriae Cocos), 12g, *Da Fu Pi* (Pericarpium arecae Catechu), 9g, *Chen Pi* (Pericarpium Citri Reticulatae), 9g, *Sheng Jiang* (uncooked Rhizoma Zingiberis), 3g

Bai Zhu San [2] (Atractylodes Powder): *Bai Zhu* (Rhizoma Atractylodis Macrocephalae), 15g, *Huang Qin* (Radix Scutellariae Baicalensis), 12g

Ban Xia Shu Mi Tang (Pinellia & Millet Decoction): *Ban Xia* (Rhizoma Pinelliae Ternatae), 10g, *Shu Mi* (Semen Panici Miliacei), 30g

Du Zhong Wan (Eucommia Pills): *Du Zhong* (Cortex Eucommiae Ulmoidis), 15g, *Xu Duan* (Radix Dipsaci), 15g

E Zhu Wan (Zedoaria Pills): *E Zhu* (Rhizoma Curcumae Zedoariae), 12g, *San Leng* (Rhizoma Sparganii), 12g, *Mu Xiang* (Radix Auklandiae Lappae), 12g, *Xiang Fu* (Rhizoma Cyperi Rotundi), 9g, *Qing Mu Xiang* (Radix Aristolochiae), 9g, *Bing Lang* (Semen Arecae Catechu), 9g, *Qian Niu Zi* (Semen Pharbiditis), 9g, *Gu Ya* (Fructus Germinatus Oryzae Sativae), 10g, *Qing Pi* (Pericarpium Citri Viride), 9g, *Bi Cheng Qie* (Fructus Cubebae), 6g, *Ding Xiang* (Flos Caryophylli), 6g

Er Dong Gao (Two Winters Syrup): *Tian Men Dong* (Tuber Asparagi Cochinensis), 12g, *Mai Men Dong* (Tuber Ophiopogonis Japonici), 12g

Er Huang San (Two Yellows Powder): *Sheng Di* (uncooked Radix Rehmanniae), 12g, *Shu Di* (cooked Radix Rehmanniae), 12g

Er Shen Wan (Two Spirits Pills): *Bu Gu Zhi* (Fructus Psoraleae Corylifoliae), 12g, *Rou Dou Kou* (Semen Myristicae Fragrantis), 12g

He Zi Tang (Terminalia Decoction): *He Zi* (Fructus Terminaliae Chebulae), 15g, *Jie Geng* (Radix Platycodi Grandiflori), 18g, *Gan Cao* (Radix Glycyrrhizae), 9g

Jie Geng Tang (Platycodon Decoction): *Gan Cao* (Radix Glycyrrhizae), 9g, Radix Platycodi Grandiflori (*Jie Geng*), 9g

Jie Geng Zhi Ke Tang (Platycodon Stop Coughing Decoction): *Jie Geng* (Radix Platycodi Grandiflori), 9g, *Zhi Ke* (Fructus Citri Aurantii), 9g

Qian Jin Bao Yun Dan (*Thousand [Pieces of] Gold* Protect Pregnancy Elixir): *Du Zhong* (Cortex Eucommiae Ulmoidis), 12g, *Xu Duan* (Radix Dipsaci), 12g, *Huang Qin* (Radix Scutellariae Bacalensis), 6g, *Bai Zhu* (Rhizoma Atractylodis Macrocephalae), 9g, *Dang Gui* (Radix Angelicae Sinensis), 9g, *Shu Di* (cooked Radix Rehmanniae), 9g, *Xiang Fu* (Rhizoma Cyperi Rotundi), 6g, *Chen Pi* (Pericarpium Citri Reticulatae), 6g, *Ren Shen* (Radix Panacis Ginseng), 6g

Xiao Ban Xia Tang (Minor Pinellia Decoction): *Ban Xia* (Rhizoma Pinelliae Ternatae), 12g, *Sheng Jiang* (uncooked Rhizoma Zingiberis), 6g

Xiao Zhong Zhi Tong Tang (Disperse Swelling & Stop Pain Decoction): *Hong Hua* (Flos Carthami Tinctorii), 9g, *Tao Ren* (Semen Pruni Persicae), 9g, *Su Mu* (Lignum Sappan), 9g, *Yan Hu Suo* (Rhizoma Corydalis Yanhusuo), 12g, *Ru Xiang* (Resina Olibani), 6g, *Mo Yao* (Resina Myrrhae), 6g, *Chi Shao* (Radix Rubrus Paeoniae Lactiflorae), 9g, *Zi Ran Tong* (Pyritum), 9g, *Chuan Xiong* (Radix Ligustici Wallichii), 12g

Xiong Gui San (Ligusticum & Dang Gui Powder): *Chuan Xiong* (Radix Ligustici Wallichii), 12g, *Dang Gui* (Radix Angelicae Sinensis), 12g

Zhen Zhong Dan (Pillow Elixir): *Yuan Zhi* (Radix Polygalae Tenuifoliae), 6g, *Shi Chang Pu* (Rhizoma Acori Graminei), 6g, *Long Gu* (Os Draconis), 15g, *Gui Ban* (Plastrum Testudinis), 15g

Zhi Zi Chi Tang (Gardenia & Soya Decoction): *Zhi Zi* (Fructus Gardeniae Jasminoidis), 9g, *Dan Dou Chi* (Semen Praeparatus Sojae), 9g

Zi Shen Wan (Enrich the Kidneys Pills): *Huang Bai* (Cortex Phellodendri), 9g, *Zhi Mu* (Rhizoma Anemarrhenae Aspheloidis), 9g, *Rou Gui* (Cortex Cinnamomi Cassiae), 3g

Bibliography

Bai Jia Pei Wu Yong Yao Jing Yan Cai Jing (The Collected Quintessence of Hundreds of Masters' Experiences in Combining Medicinals) Xiao Sen-mao & Peng Yong-kai, Chinese National Chinese Medicine & Medicinals Press, Beijing, 1992

Chang Yong Zhong Yao Chu Fang Ming Bian Yi (Discriminating the Meaning of the Names of Commonly Used Chinese Medicinals & Formulas), Xu Guo-long *et al.*, Anhui Science & Technology Press, Hefei, 1982

Jian Ming Zhong Yi Ci Dian (Concise Dictionary of Chinese Medicine), Li Yong-chun *et al.*, People's Health & Hygiene Press, Beijing, 1979

Lin Chuang Shi Yong Yao Xue (A Study of Clinically Practical Chinese Medicinals), Yan Zheng-hua *et al.*, People's Health & Hygiene Press, Beijing, 1992

Pao Zhi: An Introduction to the Use of Processed Chinese Medicinals, Philippe Sionneau, trans. by Bob Flaws, Blue Poppy press, Boulder, CO, 1995

Pharmacopee Chinoise & Acupuncture: Les Prescriptions Efficaces, Philippe Sionneau, Guy Tredaniel Editeur, Paris, 1996

Shi Jin Mo Dui Yao Lin Chuang Jing Yan Ji (A Compilation of Contemporary Knowledge & Clinical Experiences of Combining Chinese Medicinals), Lu Jing-shan, Shanxi People's Press, Taiyuan, 1982

Shi Yong Chu Fang Gang Mu (An Outline of Practical Formulas), He Lun, Shanxi Science & Technology Press, Xian, 1991

Shi Yong Du Xing Zhong Yao Xue (A Practical Study of Toxic Chinese Medicinals), Yang Fen-ming & Zeng Li-chun, Science, Technology & Literature Press, Beijing, 1992

Zhong Hua Ming Yi Fang Ji Da Quan (A Great Compendium of Famous Chinese Doctors' Formulas), Peng Huai-ren *et al.*, Jin Dun Press, Beijing, 1990

Zhong Yao Da Ci Dian (Dictionary of Chinese Materia Medica), Jiangsu College of New Medicine, Shanghai Science & Technology Press, Shanghai, 1992

Zhong Yao De Pei Wu Yun Yong (The Application of Chinese Medicinal Combinations), Ding Guang-di, People's Health & Hygiene Press, Beijing, 1982

Zhong Yao Lin Chuang Sheng Yong Yu Zhi Yong (The Clinical Use of Uncooked & Processed Chinese Medicinals), Liu Zheng, People's Health & Hygiene Press, Beijing, 1983

Zhong Yao Pao Zhi Yu Lin Chuang Ying Yong (The Clinical Application of Processed Chinese Medicinals), Hu Chang-jiang *et al.*, Sichuan Science & Technology Press, Chengdu, 1992

Zhong Yao Xing Yong Lei Bi Bian Yi (Discussions on the Discrimination of Differences Between the Uses of Chinese Medicinals of a Similar Nature), Li Xue-guo, Knowledge Center Press, Beijing, 1991

Zhong Yao Xue (A Study of Chinese Medicinals), Lin Tong-guo *et al.*, Hunan Science & Technology Press, Changsha, 1985

Zhong Yi Da Ci Dian, Zhong Yao Fen Ce (Encyclopedia of Chinese Medicine, Volume on Chinese Medicinals), People's Health & Hygiene Press, Beijing, 1982

Zhong Yi Fang Ji Ti Jie (Explanations of Chinese Medical Formulas), Jiang Ping-an, Jiangxi Science & Technology Press, Nanchang, 1985

Zhong Yi Lin Chuang Chang Yong Dui Yao Pei Wu (Clinically & Commonly Used Combinations of Medicinals in Chinese Medicine), Su Qing-ying, People's Health & Hygiene Press, Beijing, 1984

General Index

blood vacuity 51-52
wind cold; wind heat 52, 53
heart 25
  diseases 62
  nourishes the 61
  tranquilizes the 6, 25
heart and kidneys, breakdown in communication 95
heart disease, coronary 62
heart fire which rises upward 97
heart pain due to qi stagnation 49
heart pain, intense 85
heart yin, damaged 15
heat toxins, severe 105
hematemesis 8, 16, 61, 91, 95
hematuria 91
hemiplegia 5
hemoptysis 16, 91, 116
hemorrhages 16, 63, 64
hepatitis 19, 49
  chronic 19
  subacute 19
hepato-biliary disorders 41
hepatomegaly 19, 27, 41
hernia inguinal 49
hiccup 68
hyperactivity due to liver yang 43
hypercholesterolemia 62, 83, 84, 120
hypertension 7, 21, 35, 58, 84, 87, 120, 123
  arterial 120
hypochondria 117

I

illness, chronic 65
impotence 97
infantile paralysis 89
infertility due to blood stasis 72
inflammations, enduring cutaneous 51
influenza 86
injuries 92, 117, 132
  traumatic 117, 132
  with pain and swelling due to blood stasis 92
insomnia 4, 15, 43, 53
  due to yin vacuity 53
intelligence, boost the 124
intestinal abscess 118
intestinal dryness 38
irritability 59, 105, 112

J, K

jaundice 88, 128, 133
joint numbness 90
joint pain 69, 88-90, 113
  due to wind, cold, and dampness 69
joints 40, 61, 90
  hot, red, swollen, painful 40, 61
  swollen 90
knee and lumbar pain 70
knees, swollen, painful 114

L

large intestine, dryness in the 129
laryngitis 28
lateral costal pain 3, 19, 45, 50, 133
legs, pain in the 89
lily disease 15
limb pain 120
limbs 21, 35, 54, 60, 63, 76, 120
  spasms and pain in the 21
  cold 54, 76
  numbness in the 60, 63, 120
  weakness in the lower 21
  weakness of the 35
lips, pale 85
liver depression qi stagnation 18
liver-stomach disharmony with qi stagnation 133
liver qi, counterflowing 19, 20
liver yang hyperactivity of 109, 120
low back, cold feeling in the 22
lumbago or lumbar pain 17, 37, 89
lumbar pain, traumatic 70
lung abscess 118
lung qi counterflow 4, 17
lungs 42, 48, 58, 108
  accumulation of phlegm in 48, 58
  drains the 58
  drying the 108
  dryness of the 108
  feeling of oppression and downward falling of the 42

M

macula, eruption of reddish 121
malaria 41
mastitis 118
measles 83
memory, loss of 25
menstrual irregularities 5, 19, 49, 51, 61
menstrual blood, dark purple 61
menstrual cycle, long 63
menstrual flow, clots in the 61, 72
menstruation 63, 114
  delayed 63
mental depression 15

mental confusion 105, 121, 128
mental-emotional tension 18
metrorrhagia 26
middle burner, supplement the 58
miscarriage, threatened 26
mouth 49, 101
  dry 49
  sugary taste in the 101
  thick feeling in the 101
mouth ulcers, chronic, recalcitrant 80
muscles (i..e., flesh) engenders 16
myalgia in the whole body 89

N, O

nasal congestion 39
nasal phlegm, turbid 39
nausea 22, 25, 26, 30, 31-34, 41, 47, 68, 71, 80, 82, 98, 99, 101, 117, 124, 125, 128
    due to cold in stomach and qi stagnation 82
neck pain, back of the 69
necrosis 114
nephritis, chronic 90
neurasthenia 15
night crying, nightmares 43
night sweats 22
nocturia 105
nodulation, scatter 32
nodules, subcutaneous 105, 114
nose, runny 39
nosebleed 91
oligomenorrhea 122
oliguria 7, 21, 113
oral ulcers 7, 28
ovarian cysts 107

P

pain, fixed, stabbing, and severe 92
palpitations 15, 24, 25, 27, 28, 33, 53, 61, 87, 111, 120
    heart 24
    severe 61
paralysis, infantile 9, 89
parasinusitis 39
parasites, intestinal 37
pelvis, 107
    masses in the 107
    piercing pain in the 107
    spasms and contractures in the 107
perspiration 5, 22, 57, 66, 73, 76, 77, 83, 86, 100, 109, 111
    absence of 86
    cold spontaneous 76
    excessive 111
    lack of 83
    light 109
    night-time 100
    profuse 77
    promotes 22
    slight 22
    spontaneous 22, 66, 73
    stopping 66
pharyngitis 28
phlegm 5, 17, 24, 30, 33, 58, 79
    difficult to expectorate 17
    profuse, purulent 79
    transforms 33
photophobia 109
postpartum abdominal pain 51
postpartum weakness 63
premature ejaculation 94
premenstrual syndrome 19
prolapse 27, 42, 65, 73, 83, 104
    of the anus 27, 42, 73, 83

rectal and uterine 65, 83, 104
    uterine 42
pruritus 61, 104
ptosis 27, 42, 65, 83
    gastric 42
    of the organs 27
pulmonary abscess 79
purpura 61

Q, R

qi 2, 26, 58, 108
    rectify the 109
    stagnation 2, 26, 61
    supplements the 2, 58
renal lithiasis 89
respiratory diseases 18
rheumatic pains or complaints 52, 86, 117
    due to wind, cold, and dampness 86
    all over the body 69
rheumatism, inflammatory 88
rhinitis 39
    allergic 39
    chronic or acute 39
rubella 61

S

salivation, abundant 101
salpingitis 107
salpingo-ovaritis 107
scars 117
scrotal pain 131
scrotum, diseases of the 49, 107
    pain radiating toward the 107
scrotum and testicles, diseases of the 107
seminal emission 17, 93, 97, 104
    due to vacuity fire 93
    due to simultaneous heart fire and kidney yang vacuity 97
sexual desire, excessive thinking about 94
shan 107
shivers 22
sinews 9, 25, 63, 88
    blood vacuity not nourishing the 63
    pain, 9
    spasms of the 25
    stiffness of the 88
sinews & bones, strengthens 70
sinusitis, frontal 39
skin eruptions 104
skin infections, pyogenic 51, 105, 119
skin rashes 83
skin which is warm to the touch 64
sleep 15, 25
    desire to 15
    disturbed 25
smell, loss of 39
sores and welling abscesses 63
spermatorrhea 104, 111
spirit 25, 77, 111, 124

arouse the 124
 hyperactivity harassing the 111
 lassitude of the 77
 quieting the 9, 25
spleen pure heat 101
splenomegaly 27
steaming bones 35, 93, 94, 122
stomach 3, 19, 31, 33, 36, 45, 80
 clamoring 80
 harmonizes the 31, 33
 pain in the 19
 rumbling noises in the 36, 46, 52, 80, 110
 disharmony 31
stomach qi 33
 supplements the 33
 stomach qi vacuity 98
stomatitis 7, 80
stones, expels 88
stools 1, 24, 36, 39, 45, 51, 56, 66, 84, 122
 dry 1, 36
 foul-smelling 56
 loose 24, 36, 39, 45, 51, 56, 66, 84, 122
strangury 74, 88
 stone 88
 with chyluria, milky, turbid urine 74
 strangury patterns 107
strength, lack of 22, 57
strep throat 28
summerheat dampness 101
sweating 1, 2, 75
sweats, night 22
swelling 16

T

taciturnity 15
tapeworms 37
tendinitis 21
tenesmus 96
testicles 49, 107
 contracture, swelling, and hardening of the 107
 diseases of the scrotum or 49
thirst 22, 109, 114, 116, 121, 127
 absence of 127
 great 115, 121
 no 22
 slight 109
thirsting & wasting 116
throat 8, 17, 28, 79, 41, 104, 112, 116
 dry 116
 inflammations 28
 itchy 17
 pain, redness, and swelling of the 28, 79
 painful, swollen 8, 104
thromboangiitis obliterans 114
tingling or numbness 55
 of the tongue 55
tinnitus 35, 43, 53
tissue, necrotic 114, 117
toe gangrene 114, 116
tongue, dry 126

tonsillitis 28
toothache 28, 68, 83, 95, 104, 121, 123, 125
traumatic injuries 92
trembling 35
 involuntary 35
 of the hands and feet 35
tremors resolves or stops 35, 73

U

ulcers 28, 51
 oral 28, 80
urethral lithiasis 102
urinary incontinence 105, 106, 111
urinary lithiasis 88
urinary tract infection 117
urination 17, 25, 37, 40, 58, 85, 93, 97, 105, 107
 clear, long 85
 cloudy, scanty 40
 disinhibits 58
 frequent 17, 105
 frequent and abundant 37
 inhibited 93
 long, clear 97
 piercingly painful 107
 pricking, painful 93
 reduces 105
urine, dark 56
uterine bleeding during pregnancy 26

V

vaginal discharge, abnormal 17, 40, 42, 105-107, 110, 111
vaginal itching, external 40
vertigo 15, 19, 83
vexation, eliminates 58
vision blurred or unclear 17, 24
visual acuity, diminished 83
voice 78
 hoarse or husky 78
 loss of 78
vomiting 3, 22
 during pregnancy 22, 98
 stops 34

W

warm disease 15
weakness in the elderly 22
weakness, postpartum 62
wheezing 58
whooping cough 18, 116
wind 22, 35, 57
 extinguish 35
 fear of 22, 57
 with expectoration of yellow, sticky, thick phlegm 67
wounds 51, 117

OTHER BOOKS ON CHINESE MEDICINE AVAILABLE FROM:
BLUE POPPY ENTERPRISES, INC.

Colorado: 3275-B Prairie Avenue, Boulder, CO 80301
For ordering 1-800-487-9296 PH. 303-447-8372 FAX 303-245-8362
California: 1725 Monrovia Ave. Unit A4, Costa Mesa, CA 92627
For ordering 1-800-293-6697 PH. 949-270-6511 FAX 949-335-7110
Email: info@bluepoppy.com Website: www.bluepoppy.com

ACUPOINT POCKET REFERENCE
by Bob Flaws
ISBN 0-936185-93-7
ISBN 978-0-936185-93-4

ACUPUNCTURE, CHINESE MEDICINE & HEALTHY
WEIGHT LOSS   Revised Edition
by Juliette Aiyana, L. Ac.
ISBN 1-891845-61-6
ISBN 978-1-891845-61-1

ACUPUNCTURE & IVF
by Lifang Liang
ISBN 0-891845-24-1
ISBN 978-0-891845-24-6

ACUPUNCTURE FOR STROKE REHABILITATION
Three Decades of Information from China
by Hoy Ping Yee Chan, et al.
ISBN 1-891845-35-7
ISBN 978-1-891845-35-2

ACUPUNCTURE PHYSICAL MEDICINE: An Acupuncture
Touchpoint Approach to the Treatment of Chronic Pain,
Fatigue, and Stress Disorders
by Mark Seem
ISBN 1-891845-13-6
ISBN 978-1-891845-13-0

ACUPUNCTURE MEDICINE: Bodymind Integration for Bodily
Distress and Mental Pain
by Mark Seem
ISBN 1-891845-70-5
ISBN 978-1-891845-70-3

AGING & BLOOD STASIS: A New Approach to TCM Geriatrics
by Yan De-xin
ISBN 0-936185-63-6
ISBN 978-0-936185-63-7

AN ACUPUNCTURISTS GUIDE TO MEDICAL RED FLAGS &
REFERRALS
by Dr. David Anzaldua, MD
ISBN 1-891845-54-3
ISBN 978-1-891845-54-3

BETTER BREAST HEALTH NATURALLY with CHINESE
MEDICINE
by Honora Lee Wolfe & Bob Flaws
ISBN 0-936185-90-2
ISBN 978-0-936185-90-3

BIOMEDICINE: A TEXTBOOK FOR PRACTITIONERS OF
ACUPUNCTURE AND ORIENTAL MEDICINE
by Bruce H. Robinson, MD Second Edition
ISBN 1-891845-62-4
ISBN 978-1-891845-62-8

THE BOOK OF JOOK: Chinese Medicinal Porridges
by Bob Flaws
ISBN 0-936185-60-6
ISBN 978-0-936185-60-0

CHANNEL DIVERGENCES Deeper Pathways of the Web
by Miki Shima and Charles Chase
ISBN 1-891845-15-2
ISBN 978-1-891845-15-4

CHINESE MEDICAL OBSTETRICS
by Bob Flaws
ISBN 1-891845-30-6
ISBN 978-1-891845-30-7

CHINESE MEDICAL PALM IS TRY: Your Health in Your Hand
by Zong Xiao-fan & Gary Liscum
ISBN 0-936185-64-3
ISBN 978-0-936185-64-4

CHINESE MEDICAL PSYCHIATRY: A Textbook and Clinical
Manual
by Bob Flaws and James Lake, MD
ISBN 1-845891-17-9
ISBN 978-1-845891-17-8

CHINESE MEDICINAL TEAS: Simple, Proven, Folk Formulas
for Common Diseases & Promoting Health
by Zong Xiao-fan & Gary Lis cum
ISBN 0-936185-76-7
ISBN 978-0-936185-76-7

CHINESE MEDICINAL WINES & ELIXIRS
by Bob Flaws Revised Edition
ISBN 0-936185-58-9
ISBN 978-0-936185-58-3

CHINESE PEDIATRIC MASSAGE THERAPY: A Parent's &
Practitioner's Guide to the Prevention & Treatment of Childhood
Illness
by Fan Ya-li
ISBN 0-936185-54-6
ISBN 978-0-936185-54-5

CHINESE SCALP ACUPUNCTURE
by Jason Jishun Hao & Linda Lingzhi Hao
ISBN 1-891845-60-8
ISBN 978-1-891845-60-4

CHINESE SELF-MASSAGE THERAPY: The Easy Way to Health
by Fan Ya-li
ISBN 0-936185-74-0
ISBN 978-0-936185-74-3

THE CLASSIC OF DIFFICULTIES: A Translation of the Nan Jing
translation by Bob Flaws
ISBN 1-891845-07-1
ISBN 978-1-891845-07-9

A CLINICIAN'S GUIDE TO USING GRANULE
EXTRACTS
by Eric Brand
ISBN 1-891845-51-9
ISBN 978-1-891845-51-2

A COMPENDIUM OF CHINESE MEDICAL MENSTRUAL
DISEASES
by Bob Flaws
ISBN 1-891845-31-4
ISBN 978-1-891845-31-4

CONCISE CHINESE MATERIA MEDICA
by Eric Brand and Nigel Wiseman
ISBN 0-912111-82-8
ISBN 978-0-912111-82-7

CONTEMPORARY GYNECOLOGY: An Integrated Chinese-
Western Approach
by Lifang Liang
ISBN 1-891845-50-0
ISBN 978-1-891845-50-5

CONTROLLING DIABETES NATURALLY WITH CHINESE
MEDICINE
by Lynn Kuchinski
ISBN 0-936185-06-3
ISBN 978-0-936185-06-2

CURING ARTHRITIS NATURALLY WITH CHINESE
MEDICINE
by Douglas Frank & Bob Flaws
ISBN 0-936185-87-2
ISBN 978-0-936185-87-3

CURING DEPRESSION NATURALLY WITH CHINESE
MEDICINE
by Rosa Schnyer & Bob Flaws
ISBN 0-936185-94-5
ISBN 978-0-936185-94-1

CURING FIBROMYALGIA NATURALLY WITH CHINESE
MEDICINE
by Bob Flaws
ISBN 1-891845-09-8
ISBN 978-1-891845-09-3

CURING HAY FEVER NATURALLY WITH CHINESE
MEDICINE
by Bob Flaws
ISBN 0-936185-91-0
ISBN 978-0-936185-91-0

CURING HEADACHES NATURALLY WITH CHINESE
MEDICINE
by Bob Flaws
ISBN 0-936185-95-3
ISBN 978-0-936185-95-8

CURING IBS NATURALLY WITH CHINESE
MEDICINE
by Jane Bean Oberski
ISBN 1-891845-11-X
ISBN 978-1-891845-11-6

CURING INSOMNIA NATURALLY WITH CHINESE
MEDICINE
by Bob Flaws
ISBN 0-936185-86-4
ISBN 978-0-936185-86-6

CURING PMS NATURALLY WITH CHINESE MEDICINE
by Bob Flaws
ISBN 0-936185-85-6
ISBN 978-0-936185-85-9

DISEASES OF THE KIDNEY & BLADDER
by Hoy Ping Yee Chan, et al.
ISBN 1-891845-37-3
ISBN 978-1-891845-35-6

THE DIVINE FARMER'S MATERIA MEDICA: A Translation of
the Shen Nong Ben Cao
translation by Yang Shouz-zhong
ISBN 0-936185-96-1
ISBN 978-0-936185-96-5

DUI YAO: THE ART OF COMBINING CHINESE HERBAL
MEDICINALS
by Philippe Sionneau
ISBN 0-936185-81-3
ISBN 978-0-936185-81-1

ENDOMETRIOSIS, INFERTILITY AND TRADITIONAL
CHINESE MEDICINE: A Layperson's Guide
by Bob Flaws
ISBN 0-936185-14-7
ISBN 978-0-936185-14-9

THE ESSENCE OF LIU FENG-WU'S GYNECOLOGY
by Liu Feng-wu, translated by Yang Shou-zhong
ISBN 0-936185-88-0
ISBN 978-0-936185-88-0

EXTRA TREATISES BASED ON INVESTIGATION &
INQUIRY: A Translation of Zhu Dan-xi's Ge Zhi Yu Lun
translation by Yang Shou-zhong
ISBN 0-936185-53-8
ISBN 978-0-936185-53-8

FIRE IN THE VALLEY: TCM Diagnosis & Treatment of Vaginal
Diseases
by Bob Flaws
ISBN 0-936185-25-2
ISBN 978-0-936185-25-5

FULFILLING THE ESSENCE:
A Handbook of Traditional & Contemporary Treatments for
Female Infertility
by Bob Flaws
ISBN 0-936185-48-1
ISBN 978-0-936185-48-4

FU QING-ZHU'S GYNECOLOGY
trans. by Yang Shou-zhong and Liu Da-wei
ISBN 0-936185-35-X
ISBN 978-0-936185-35-4

GOLDEN NEEDLE WANG LE-TING: A 20th Century Master's
Approach to Acupuncture
by Yu Hui-chan and Han Fu-ru, trans. by Shuai Xue-zhong
ISBN 0-936185-78-3
ISBN 978-0-936185-78-1

A HANDBOOK OF CHINESE HEMATOLOGY
by Simon Becker
ISBN 1-891845-16-0
ISBN 978-1-891845-16-1

A HANDBOOK OF TCM PATTERNS & THEIR TREATMENTS
Second Edition
by Bob Flaws & Daniel Finney
ISBN 0-936185-70-8
ISBN 978-0-936185-70-5

A HANDBOOK OF TRADITIONAL CHINESE DERMATOLOGY
by Liang Jian-hui, trans. by Zhang Ting-liang
& Bob Flaws
ISBN 0-936185-46-5
ISBN 978-0-936185-46-0

A HANDBOOK OF TRADITIONAL CHINESE GYNECOLOGY
by Zhejiang College of TCM, trans. by Zhang Ting-liang
& Bob Flaws
ISBN 0-936185-06-6 (4th edit.)
ISBN 978-0-936185-06-4

A HANDBOOK of TCM PEDIATRICS
by Bob Flaws
ISBN 0-936185-72-4
ISBN 978-0-936185-72-9

THE HEART & ESSENCE OF DAN-XI'S METHODS OF
TREATMENT
by Xu Dan-xi, trans. by Yang Shou-zhong
ISBN 0-926185-50-3
ISBN 978-0-936185-50-7

HERB TOXICITIES & DRUG INTERACTIONS:
A Formula Approach
by Fred Jennes with Bob Flaws
ISBN 1-891845-26-8
ISBN 978-1-891845-26-0

IMPERIAL SECRETS OF HEALTH & LONGEVITY
by Bob Flaws
ISBN 0-936185-51-1
ISBN 978-0-936185-51-4

INSIGHTS OF A SENIOR ACUPUNCTURIST
by Miriam Lee
ISBN 0-936185-33-3
ISBN 978-0-936185-33-0

INTEGRATED PHARMACOLOGY: Combining Modern
Pharmacology with Chinese Medicine
by Dr. Greg Sperber with Bob Flaws
ISBN 1-891845-41-1
ISBN 978-0-936185-41-3

INTEGRATIVE PHARMACOLOGY: Combining Modern
Pharmacology with Integrative Medicine   Second Edition
by Dr. Greg Sperber with Bob Flaws
ISBN 1-891845-69-1
ISBN 978-0-936185-69-7

INTRODUCTION TO THE USE OF PROCESSED CHINESE
MEDICINALS
by Philippe Sionneau
ISBN 0-936185-62-7
ISBN 978-0-936185-62-0

KEEPING YOUR CHILD HEALTHY WITH CHINESE
MEDICINE
by Bob Flaws
ISBN 0-936185-71-6
ISBN 978-0-936185-71-2

THE LAKESIDE MASTER'S STUDY OF THE PULSE
by Li Shi-zhen, trans. by Bob Flaws
ISBN 1-891845-01-2
ISBN 978-1-891845-01-7

MANAGING MENOPAUSE NATURALLY WITH CHINESE
MEDICINE
by Honora Lee Wolfe
ISBN 0-936185-98-8
ISBN 978-0-936185-98-9

MASTER HUA'S CLASSIC OF THE CENTRAL VISCERA
by Hua Tuo, trans. by Yang Shou-zhong
ISBN 0-936185-43-0
ISBN 978-0-936185-43-9

THE MEDICAL I CHING: Oracle of the Healer Within
by Miki Shima
ISBN 0-936185-38-4
ISBN 978-0-936185-38-5

MENOPAIUSE & CHINESE MEDICINE
by Bob Flaws
ISBN 1-891845-40-3
ISBN 978-1-891845-40-6

MOXIBUSTION: A MODERN CLINICAL HANDBOOK
by Lorraine Wilcox
ISBN 1-891845-49-7
ISBN 978-1-891845-49-9

MOXIBUSTION: THE POWER OF MUGWORT FIRE
by Lorraine Wilcox
ISBN 1-891845-46-2
ISBN 978-1-891845-46-8

A NEW AMERICAN ACUPUNTURE By Mark Seem
ISBN 0-936185-44-9
ISBN 978-0-936185-44-6

PLAYING THE GAME: A Step-by-Step Approach to Accepting
Insurance as an Acupuncturist
by Greg Sperber & Tiffany Anderson-Hefner
ISBN 3-131416-11-7
ISBN 978-3-131416-11-7

POCKET ATLAS OF CHINESE MEDICINE
Edited by Marne and Kevin Ergil
ISBN 1-891-845-59-4
ISBN 978-1-891845-59-8

POINTS FOR PROFIT: The Essential Guide to Practice Success
for Acupuncturists   5th Fully Edited Edition
by Honora Wolfe with Marilyn Allen
ISBN 1-891845-25-X
ISBN 978-1-891845-25-3

PRINCIPLES OF CHINESE MEDICAL ANDROLOGY: An
Integrated Approach to Male Reproductive and Urological
Health by Bob Damone
ISBN 1-891845-45-4
ISBN 978-1-891845-45-1

PRINCE WEN HUI's COOK: Chinese Dietary Therapy
by Bob Flaws & Honora Wolfe
ISBN 0-912111-05-4
ISBN 978-0-912111-05-6

THE PULSE CLASSIC: A Translation of the Mai Jing
by Wang Shu-he, trans. by Yang Shou-zhong
ISBN 0-936185-75-9
ISBN 978-0-936185-75-0

THE SECRET OF CHINESE PULSE DIAGNOSIS by Bob Flaws
ISBN 0-936185-67-8
ISBN 978-0-936185-67-5

SECRET SHAOLIN FORMULAS FOR THE TREATMENT OF
EXTERNAL INJURY
by De Chan, trans. by Zhang Ting-liang & Bob Flaws
ISBN 0-936185-08-2
ISBN 978-0-936185-08-8

STATEMENTS OF FACT IN TRADITIONAL CHINESE MEDICINE
by Bob Flaws   Revised & Expanded
ISBN 0-936185-52-X
ISBN 978-0-936185-52-1

STICKING TO THE POINT: A Step-by-Step Approach to TCM
Acupuncture Therapy
by Bob Flaws & Honora Wolfe 2 Condensed Books
ISBN 1-891845-47-0
ISBN 978-1-891845-47-5

A STUDY OF DAOIST ACUPUNCTURE
by Liu Zheng-cai
ISBN 1-891845-08-X
ISBN 978-1-891845-08-6

THE SUCCESSFUL CHINESE HERBALIST
by Bob Flaws and Honora Lee Wolfe
ISBN 1-891845-29-2
ISBN 978-1-891845-29-1

THE SYSTEMATIC CLASSIC OF ACUPUNCTURE &
MOXIBUSTION: A translation of the Jia Yi Jing
by Huang-fu Mi, trans. by Yang Shou-zhong & Charles Chace
ISBN 0-936185-29-5
ISBN 978-0-936185-29-3

THE TAO OF HEALTHY EATING: DIETARY
WISDOM ACCORDING TO CHINESE MEDICINE
by Bob Flaws Second Edition
ISBN 0-936185-92-9
ISBN 978-0-936185-92-7

TEACH YOURSELF TO READ MODERN MEDICAL CHINESE
by Bob Flaws
ISBN 0-936185-99-6
ISBN 978-0-936185-99-6

TEST PREP WORKBOOK FOR BASIC TCM THEORY
by Zhong Bai-song
ISBN 1-891845-43-8
ISBN 978-1-891845-43-7

TEST PREP WORKBOOK FOR THE NCCAOM BIOMEDICINE
MODULE: Exam Preparation & Study Guide
by Zhong Bai-song
ISBN 1-891845-34-9
ISBN 978-1-891845-34-5

TREATING PEDIATRIC BED-WETTING WITH ACUPUNCTURE
& CHINESE MEDICINE
by Robert Helmer
ISBN 1-891845-33-0
ISBN 978-1-891845-33-8

TREATISE on the SPLEEN & STOMACH: A Translation and
annotation of Li Dong-yuan's Pi Wei Lun
by Bob Flaws
ISBN 0-936185-41-4
ISBN 978-0-936185-41-5

THE TREATMENT OF CARDIOVASCULAR DISEASES WITH
CHINESE MEDICINE
by Simon Becker, Bob Flaws & Robert Casañas, MD
ISBN 1-891845-27-6
ISBN 978-1-891845-27-7

THE TREATMENT OF DIABETES MELLITUS WITH CHINESE
MEDICINE
by Bob Flaws, Lynn Kuchinski & Robert Casañas, M.D.
ISBN 1-891845-21-7
ISBN 978-1-891845-21-5

THE TREATMENT OF DISEASE IN TCM, Vol. 1: Diseases of
the Head & Face, Including Mental & Emotional Disorders New
Edition
by Philippe Sion neau & Lü Gang
ISBN 0-936185-69-4
ISBN 978-0-936185-69-9

THE TREATMENT OF DISEASE IN TCM, Vol. II:
Diseases of the Eyes, Ears, Nose, & Throat
by Sionneau & Lü
ISBN 0-936185-73-2
ISBN 978-0-936185-73-6

THE TREATMENT OF DISEASE IN TCM, Vol. III: Diseases of
the Mouth, Lips, Tongue, Teeth & Gums
by Sionneau & Lü
ISBN 0-936185-79-1
ISBN 978-0-936185-79-8

THE TREATMENT OF DISEASE IN TCM, Vol IV: Diseases of
the Neck, Shoulders, Back, & Limbs
by Phi lippe Sion neau & Lü Gang
ISBN 0-936185-89-9
ISBN 978-0-936185-89-7

THE TREATMENT OF DISEASE IN TCM, Vol V: Diseases of
the Chest & Abdomen
by Philippe Sionneau & Lü Gang
ISBN 1-891845-02-0
ISBN 978-1-891845-02-4

THE TREATMENT OF DISEASE IN TCM, Vol VI: Diseases of
the Urogential System & Proctology
by Phi lippe Sion neau & Lü Gang
ISBN 1-891845-05-5
ISBN 978-1-891845-05-5

THE TREATMENT OF DISEASE IN TCM, Vol VII:
General Symptoms
by Phi lippe Sion neau & Lü Gang
ISBN 1-891845-14-4
ISBN 978-1-891845-14-7

THE TREATMENT OF EXTER NAL DIS EASES WITH
ACUPUNCTURE & MOXIBUSTION
by Yan Cui-lan and Zhu Yun-long, trans. by Yang Shou-zhong
ISBN 0-936185-80-5
ISBN 978-0-936185-80-4

THE TREATMENT OF MODERN WESTERN
MEDICAL DISEASES WITH CHINESE MEDICINE
by Bob Flaws & Philippe Sionneau
ISBN 1-891845-20-9
ISBN 978-1-891845-20-8

UNDERSTANDING THE DIFFICULT PATIENT: A Guide for
Practitioners of Oriental Medicine
by Nancy Bilello, RN, L.ac.
ISBN 1-891845-32-2
ISBN 978-1-891845-32-1

WESTERN PHYSICAL EXAM SKILLS FOR PRACTITIONERS
OF ASIAN MEDICINE
by Bruce H. Robinson & Honora Lee Wolfe
ISBN 1-891845-48-9
ISBN 978-1-891845-48-2

YI LIN GAI CUO (Correcting the Errors in the Forest of
Medicine)
by Wang Qing-ren
ISBN 1-891845-39-X
ISBN 978-1-891845-39-0

70 ESSENTIAL CHINESE HERBAL FORMULAS
by Bob Flaws
ISBN 0-936185-59-7
ISBN 978-0-936185-59-0

160 ESSENTIAL CHINESE READY-MADE MEDICINES
by Bob Flaws
ISBN 1-891945-12-8
ISBN 978-1-891945-12-3

630 QUESTIONS & ANSWERS ABOUT CHINESE HERBAL
MEDICINE:
A Work book & Study Guide
by Bob Flaws
ISBN 1-891845-04-7
ISBN 978-1-891845-04-8

260 ESSENTIAL CHINESE MEDICINALS
by Bob Flaws
ISBN 1-891845-03-9
ISBN 978-1-891845-03-1

750 QUESTIONS & ANSWERS ABOUT ACUPUNCTURE
Exam Preparation & Study Guide
by Fred Jennes
ISBN 1-891845-22-5
ISBN 978-1-891845-22-2